Disorders of Fat and Cellulite

SERIES IN COSMETIC AND LASER THERAPY

Series Editors
David J. Goldberg, Nicholas J. Lowe, and Gary P. Lask
Published in association with the Journal of Cosmetic and Laser Therapy

David J. Goldberg, *Fillers in Cosmetic Dermatology*, ISBN 9781841845098
Philippe Deprez, *Textbook of Chemical Peels*, ISBN 9781841842954
C. William Hanke, Gerhard Sattler, Boris Sommer, *Textbook of Liposuction*, ISBN 9781841845326
Paul J. Carniol, Neil S. Sadick, *Clinical Procedures in Laser Skin Rejuvenation*, ISBN 9780415414135
David J. Goldberg, *Laser Hair Removal*, Second Edition, ISBN 9780415414128
Benjamin Ascher, Marina Landau, Bernard Rossi, *Injection Treatments in Cosmetic Surgery*, ISBN 9780415386517
Avi Shai, Robert Baran, Howard I. Maibach, *Handbook of Cosmetic Skin Care*, Second Edition, ISBN 9780415467186
Jenny Kim, Gary Lask, *Comprehensive Aesthetic Rejuvenation: A Regional Approach*, ISBN 9780415458948
Paul Carniol, Gary Monheit, *Aesthetic Rejuvenation Challenges and Solutions: A Global Perspective*, ISBN 9780415475600
Neil Sadick, Diane Berson, Mary P. Lupo, Zoe Diana Draelos, Cosmeceutical Science in Clinical Practice, ISBN 9780415471145
Anthony Benedetto, *Botulinum Toxins in Clinical Aesthetic Practice*, Second Edition, ISBN 9780415476362
Robert Baran, Howard I. Maibach, *Textbook of Cosmetic Dermatology*, Fourth Edition, ISBN 9781841847009
David J. Goldberg, Alexander L. Berlin, *Disorders of Fat and Cellulite: Advances in Diagnosis and Treatment*, ISBN 9780415477000
Kenneth Beer, Mary P. Lupo, Vic A. Narurkar, *Cosmetic Bootcamp Primer: Comprehensive Aesthetic Management*, ISBN 9781841846989
Neil S. Sadick, Paul J. Carniol, Deborshi Roy, Luitgard Wiest, *Illustrated Manual of Injectable Fillers: A Technical Guide to the Volumetric Approach to Whole Body Rejuvenation*, ISBN 9780415476447

Disorders of Fat and Cellulite

Advances in Diagnosis and Treatment

Edited by

David J. Goldberg, M.D., J.D.
Department of Dermatology
Mt. Sinai School of Medicine
New York, New York
Fordham University School of Law
New York, New York
Skin Laser and Surgery Specialists of New York
and New Jersey, New York

Alexander L. Berlin, M.D.
U.S. Dermatology Medical Group
Arlington, Texas
Division of Dermatology
New Jersey Medical School
Newark, New Jersey

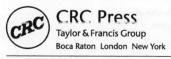

CRC Press
Taylor & Francis Group
Boca Raton London New York

CRC Press is an imprint of the
Taylor & Francis Group, an **informa** business

CRC Press
Taylor & Francis Group
6000 Broken Sound Parkway NW, Suite 300
Boca Raton, FL 33487-2742

First issued in paperback 2017

A CIP record for this book is available from the British Library.

ISBN-13: 978-0-415-47700-0 (hbk)
ISBN-13: 978-1-138-11466-1 (pbk)
ISSN (print): 2158-0286
ISSN (online): 2158-026X

Visit the Taylor & Francis Web site at
http://www.taylorandfrancis.com

and the CRC Press Web site at
http://www.crcpress.com

Library of Congress Cataloging-in-Publication Data

Disorders of fat and cellulite : advances in diagnosis and treatment / edited by David J. Goldberg, Alexander L. Berlin.
    p. ; cm. -- (Series in cosmetic and laser therapy)
  Includes bibliographical references and index.

  ISBN 978-0-415-47700-0 (hb : alk. paper) 1. Adipose tissues--Surgery. 2. Adipose tissues--Pathophysiology. 3. Adipose tissues--Physiology. 4. Cellulite. 5. Surgery, Plastic. I. Goldberg, David J., M.D. II. Berlin, Alexander L. III. Series: Series in cosmetic and laser therapy.

  [DNLM: 1. Adipose Tissue--physiology. 2. Adipose Tissue--surgery. 3. Obesity--surgery. 4. Reconstructive Surgical Procedures. QS 532.5.A3]
  RD119.5.L55D57 2011
  617.9'52--dc23

                           2011021176

For corporate sales please contact: CorporateBooksIHC@informa.com
For foreign rights please contact: RightsIHC@informa.com
For reprint permissions please contact: PermissionsIHC@informa.com

Typeset by MPS Limited, a Macmillan Company.
Printed and bound in the United Kingdom.

Contents

Contributors

Robert Anolik   Laser & Skin Surgery Center of New York, New York, New York, U.S.A.

Javad Beheshti   Division of Dermatopathology, University of Texas Southwestern Medical Center, Dallas, Texas, U.S.A.

Alexander L. Berlin   U.S. Dermatology Medical Group, Arlington, Texas; and Division of Dermatology, New Jersey Medical School, Newark, New Jersey, U.S.A.

Lori Brightman   Laser & Skin Surgery Center of New York, New York, New York, U.S.A.

Kimberly Butterwick   Cosmetic Laser Dermatology, San Diego, California, U.S.A.

Jennifer Chwalek   Skin Laser and Surgery Specialists of New York and New Jersey, Hackensack, New Jersey, U.S.A.

Clay J. Cockerell   Division of Dermatopathology, University of Texas Southwestern Medical Center, Dallas, Texas, U.S.A.

Wael A. Ghattas   South Shore Dermatology and Laser, Boston, Massachusetts, U.S.A.

David J. Goldberg   Department of Dermatology, Mt. Sinai School of Medicine, New York; Fordham University School of Law, New York; and Skin Laser and Surgery Specialists of New York and New Jersey, New York, U.S.A.

Pritesh S. Karia   Mohs and Dermatologic Surgery Center, Department of Dermatology, Dana Farber Cancer Institute/Brigham and Women's Hospital, Harvard Medical School, Boston, Massachusetts, U.S.A.

Bruce E. Katz Juva Skin & Laser Center, and Cosmetic Surgery & Laser Clinic, Mt. Sinai Medical Center, New York, New York, U.S.A.

W. Clark Lambert Department of Pathology and Division of Dermatology, New Jersey Medical School, Newark, New Jersey, U.S.A.

Naomi Lawrence Division of Dermatology, Cooper University Hospital, Marlton, New Jersey, U.S.A.

Margarita Lolis Division of Dermatology, New Jersey Medical School, Newark, New Jersey, U.S.A.

Jason Marquart Division of Dermatology, Cooper University Hospital, Marlton, New Jersey, U.S.A.

Jason C. McBean Private Practice, Fairfield, Connecticut, U.S.A.

Andrei I. Metelitsa Division of Dermatology, University of Calgary, Calgary, Alberta, Canada

Ron Overberg Nutriwellness; Environmental Health Center–Dallas, Dallas, Texas, U.S.A.

Andriy Pavlenko Division of Dermatology, New Jersey Medical School, Newark, New Jersey, U.S.A.

Jaggi Rao Division of Dermatology, University of Calgary, Calgary, Alberta, Canada

Adam M. Rotunda David Geffen School of Medicine, University of California at Los Angeles, Los Angeles, California, U.S.A.

Chrysalyne D. Schmults Mohs and Dermatologic Surgery Center, Department of Dermatology, Dana Farber Cancer Institute/Brigham and Women's Hospital, Harvard Medical School, Boston, Massachusetts, U.S.A.

Robert A. Schwartz Division of Dermatology, New Jersey Medical School, Newark, New Jersey, U.S.A.

Preface

In addition to performing multiple physiological functions in the body, subcutaneous adipose tissue provides support for the overlying skin and thus greatly contributes to the overall shape of the body. As a result, alterations in the amount of subcutaneous fat lead to significant changes in appearance. Numerous techniques have been developed over the years to deal with abnormalities of adipose tissue—both excess, as seen in obesity, and loss of fat, most commonly encountered in facial lipodystrophy associated with the aging process.

As the number of techniques, devices, and available injectable materials has increased tremendously in the last several years, so has our understanding of the normal and pathological processes occurring in this part of the body. Thus, a book designed to incorporate the current knowledge of physiology of fat and the numerous treatment modalities available today has become essential.

In the ensuing chapters, the reader is presented with the most current and complete review of the anatomy, physiology, and pathophysiology of fat and cellulite and the most up-to-date discussion of treatments and procedures available for the disorders of adipose tissue. Invaluable pearls from the authoritative figures in their respective fields will enhance any medical or cosmetic practice. Separate chapters address diet and exercise as adjunctive, yet essential, modalities and potential legal issues and ramifications of using the latest cosmetic therapies. In addition, clear figures, patient photographs, and informative tables enhance the visual aspect of the presented material, allowing the reader to examine clinical evidence behind each treatment modality.

David J. Goldberg
Alexander L. Berlin

1

Anatomy and adipogenesis

Margarita Lolis, Andriy Pavlenko, Robert A. Schwartz, and W. Clark Lambert

INTRODUCTION

Adipose tissue, or fat, is a loose connective tissue that serves many purposes, both structural and functional, in the body. It is primarily composed of adipocytes, or fat-containing cells, as well as leukocytes, macrophages, blood vessels, and fibroblastic cells, which are all held together in an array of collagen fibers. There are two forms of adipose tissue in mammals: white adipose tissue, which forms most adult adipose tissue, and brown adipose tissue.

Although adipose tissue is mainly involved in lipid anabolism, storage, and catabolism, it has also been implicated in a number of physiological and endocrine processes. Structurally, fat insulates and cushions organs to protect them from mechanical forces. Functionally, it regulates energy metabolism through lipogenesis and lipolysis, produces hormones and cytokines—often referred to as adipokines—such as leptin, resistin, and TNF-α, and mediates insulin regulation, inflammation, and cancer (1–6).

Adipogenesis is a complex and highly regulated process thought to be mediated by a variety of genes in pluripotent stem cells (Fig. 1.1) (7–9). It occurs de novo in various anatomic sites, predominantly in subcutaneous layers of the skin, and also around the heart, kidneys, and other organs (7). These specific locations of fat are known as "adipose depots." Each adipose depot has its own microenvironment composed of different cytokines and adipokines (10,11).

BACKGROUND

Obesity has become a pandemic, particularly among Western countries. The ramifications of this disease are so extensive that they have penetrated many political and economic arenas and have fueled much biological research.

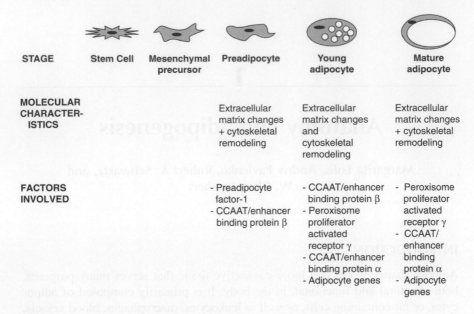

STAGE	Stem Cell	Mesenchymal precursor	Preadipocyte	Young adipocyte	Mature adipocyte
MOLECULAR CHARACTER-ISTICS			Extracellular matrix changes + cytoskeletal remodeling	Extracellular matrix changes and cytoskeletal remodeling	Extracellular matrix changes + cytoskeletal remodeling
FACTORS INVOLVED			- Preadipocyte factor-1 - CCAAT/enhancer binding protein β	- CCAAT/enhancer binding protein β - Peroxisome proliferator activated receptor γ - CCAAT/enhancer binding protein α - Adipocyte genes	- Peroxisome proliferator activated receptor γ - CCAAT/ enhancer binding protein α - Adipocyte genes

Figure 1.1 Adipocyte differentiation process.

Understanding adipogenesis, the formation of adipose tissue at the molecular and cellular level, will eventually provide the key to future antiobesity therapy and is already forming the foundation for advances within the dermatologic, medical, surgical, and cosmetic fields (12–14).

Originally, adipocytes were viewed as passive structures. Their main role in lipid homeostasis was presumed to be in the storage of energy in the form of triacylglycerol and in its release in the form of free fatty acids and glycerol. This view has evolved to one of an active, multifunctional organ. Adipose tissue is involved in the regulation of insulin resistance, vascular disease, immunological responses, and energy balance (6). Adipocytes are also involved in endocrine and paracrine functions. An example of this function is leptin. Leptin is produced by adipocytes and is then secreted into the bloodstream. It targets the hypothalamus, where it suppresses appetite and increases energy use. In a paracrine fashion, leptin also acts locally to regulate metabolism and other cellular functions. In addition, multiple other factors produced by fat cells are involved in energy regulation and homeostasis (1,4,6,15,16). These factors are explored in more detail in the next chapter.

In the past, scientists believed that humans were born with a certain number of adipocytes or that these cells developed early on after birth and did not change throughout life. This erroneous notion was called the "fixed adipocyte number" and determined whether someone was lean or obese (17). Instead, we now know that adipocytes undergo hypertrophy and hyperplasia and that these processes continue throughout life (6,18). During adipogenesis, preadipocytes proliferate and differentiate into mature adipocytes. This process is mainly activated when there is a net increase in calories (16,19–21). This current view of adipogenesis has revolutionized our view of adipocyte tissue as one that is a dynamic structure, with the preadipocyte being central to its growth, function, and distribution.

CURRENT STATE OF KNOWLEDGE

Histology of Adipose Tissue

Adipose tissue is composed of many cell types including adipocytes, preadipocytes, fibroblasts, endothelial cells, macrophages, and multipotent stem cells. Mature adipocytes comprise approximately one-third of fat tissue, whereas the remaining two-thirds are composed of small blood vessels, nerves, preadipocytes, and fibroblasts (22). There are two types of adipose tissue, white and brown.

White Adipose Tissue

Grossly, adipose tissue is a yellow, homogenous structure with finely divided septae and a glistening surface. Microscopically, white adipocytes contain one large droplet of triglycerides, which comprises 85% of the cell volume. The small nucleus and cytoplasm constitute the remaining 15% of cell volume. Thus, white adipose tissue is characteristically unilocular, with signet-ring–shaped cells ranging from 25 to 200 μm in size (Fig. 1.2) (3).

Ultrastructurally, adipocytes differ depending on the stage of maturation of each fat cell. Preadipocytes, or developing adipocytes, are typically spindle shaped and have a high content of endoplasmic reticulum and small mitochondria. During maturation, lipid accumulates as small perinuclear inclusions, which coalesce to form larger lipid droplets, the mitochondria become filamentous, and the endoplasmic reticulum becomes less prominent. Once mature, the lipid droplet occupies nearly the entirety of the cell, flattening the nucleus against the cytoplasmic membrane. Adjacent to the cell membrane are foci of basement membrane, which are closely opposed to capillaries. Although white adipose tissue is not heavily vascularized, each adipocyte is supplied by at least one capillary for support of its active metabolism. Rarely, nerves may run along the collagenous septae (3,19).

Historically, the function of white adipose tissue was thought to be for energy storage. However, its role as an endocrine organ has recently come to light. White adipocytes secrete many hormones, called adipokines, which are involved in metabolism, inflammation, and insulin regulation (22).

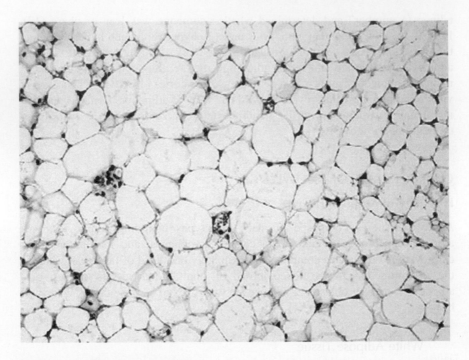

Figure 1.2 White adipose tissue.

Brown Adipose Tissue

Brown adipose tissue is predominant in newborns and hibernating animals (23). Grossly, it appears brown because of its high content of mitochondria and rich vascularization. Structurally, brown fat cells differ from white fat cells in that they are multilocular. Thus, instead of one large lipid droplet, they contain several smaller droplets, which accounts for the generally smaller size of brown adipocytes—approximately 60 μm in diameter (Fig. 1.3) (3).

As discussed in the preceding text, brown adipocytes are rich in mitochondria, whose main function in this tissue is the generation of heat, or thermogenesis. In the process, fat molecules are first broken down into fatty acids and then metabolized in the mitochondria. With the help of an uncoupling protein, thermogenin, the energy is released directly as heat. This process is discussed in greater detail in the next chapter.

Development of Subcutaneous Fat

The embryologic development of the hypodermis, where the majority of adipose tissue is located, is well understood. By day 50 to 60 of embryonic gestational age, the hypodermis has developed and is separated from the overlying dermis

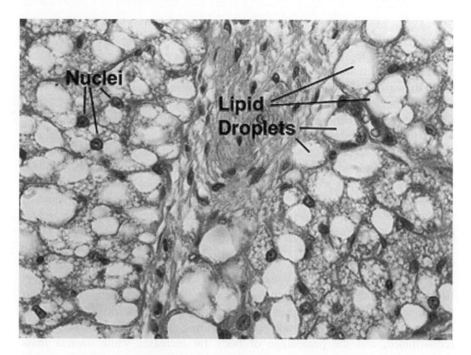

Figure 1.3 Brown adipose tissue.

by a plane of vessels. By the end of the first trimester, histological differences between the dermis and hypodermis become evident. During the second trimester, preadipocytes develop and form lipids. By the third trimester, the pre-adipocytes have matured into adipocytes and the hypodermis has become organized into fat lobules separated by fibrous septae (24).

Body Fat Distribution

Body fat distribution is multifactorial. Genetics account for roughly 30% to 50% of variability in body fat. Age, gender, physical activity, and nutritional habits are additional factors. More specifically, differences in regional fat distribution between men and women are related to hormone activity. The gynoid habitus or "pear distribution" is classically associated with the female shape and it is characterized by the presence of subcutaneous fat mostly in the trochanteric area. Its regional distribution is influenced by estrogen and progesterone, which stimulate accumulation of fat subcutaneously and decrease fat viscerally. Subcutaneous fat also has more estrogen receptors than testosterone receptors (25). By contrast, the "android" shape of men is described as fat primarily distributed viscerally or intra-abdominally. This type of adipose tissue has higher expression of androgen receptors (25). This difference in fat distribution may be because of lipoprotein lipase (LPL) activity. This enzyme regulates the uptake of fatty acids and fat accumulation. Higher activity of LPL has been found in men and is associated with the development of intra-abdominal fat. Visceral adiposity has been shown to be an independent risk factor for cardiovascular disease (25). Subcutaneous fat, on the other hand, does not have as high levels of LPL as visceral fat, and therefore less visceral obesity is seen in women.

Body fat distribution, rather than total body fat, has been associated with metabolic and cardiovascular disorders, specifically the metabolic syndrome (25–27). The android body type, where fat is mostly stored centrally and viscerally, is associated with cardiovascular disease, as opposed to the gynoid habitus, which has a lower prevalence of such diseases. This may be because of the fact that visceral adipose tissue is known to secrete interleukins, vascular endothelial growth factor (VEGF), and plasminogen activator inhibitor-1, which have all been implicated in heart disease. This is discussed in more detail in the next chapter.

Aside from body fat distribution, the percentage of body fat also differs between men and women. Overall, women have a higher percentage of body fat than men, and they mostly gain fat during puberty. In contrast, the body fat content of men peaks in early adolescence. During the aging process, body fat is redistributed, and the percentage of body fat increases while muscle mass declines (3).

Adipogenesis

The current model of adipogenesis has been derived from cumulative and comparative data using both clonal and primary preadipocyte cell lines. A breakthrough in adipocyte research came about when the first preadipocytes were cloned from Swiss 3T3 mouse embryos by two scientists, Green and Kehinde (28). From these, many cell lines were grown for further research on adipogenesis. These cell lines were composed of unipotent preadipocytes, which had already undergone determination but not differentiation. These cells are ideal to study adipogenesis because they can remain as preadipocytes or undergo differentiation following induction with various agents (28–30).

Adipogenesis has primarily been studied in vitro. The study of adipogenesis in vivo is arduous, as there are anatomic as well as unique hormonal differences among fat deposits within the body (30). More specifically, preadipocytes originating from different anatomic locations vary their response to adipogenic stimulation. In vitro studies investigating differences in adipocyte differentiation from various anatomic sites have broadened our understanding of how fat depots may have different impact on one's health (31,32).

The first step in the adipogenesis is determination. During embryonic development, pluripotent precursor stem cells become multipotent mesenchymal stem cells (MSCs) which have the capability of differentiation into various tissues, such as adipose tissue, cartilage, bone, and muscle (20,21). Subsequently, these MSCs are channeled to become adipocytes through the process of determination, which has yet to be fully elucidated. During this process, fibroblastic-appearing preadipocytes are created and committed toward adipocyte differentiation. This differentiation begins during embryonic development and finishes after birth (18,33). Once the initial event of adipocyte differentiation has occurred, one reserves the capability of forming mature adipocytes from preadipocytes throughout life when necessary (18,34). Other species do not undergo differentiation during gestation and only begin this process after birth. It is believed that humans have developed this capability to effectively use fat stores during times of deprivation.

Preadipocytes have been widely studied since the advent of immortal cell lines. Since they lack a molecular marker, preadipocytes are defined by their commitment to the adipocyte lineage and by their similarity to fibroblasts. Morphologically, they are similar to fibroblasts in that if they are coated on the bottom of a culture plate, they form a monolayer. Once a monolayer is formed, each cell contacts its neighbor, which results in growth arrest at the G1/S cell cycle phase through contact inhibition. The growth arrest is one of the most critical processes, as it commits the preadipocyte to terminal differentiation (18,27). It is not only the first step in this pathway, but is also a required one, as preadipocytes cannot differentiate into mature adipocytes if they have not entered the growth arrest phase (6). In contrast, confluence is not required, as shown in experiments where preadipocytes are plated at low density in serum-free medium or are kept in a methylcellulose suspension and still undergo differentiation (35,36).

Following confluence and growth arrest, preadipocytes must receive an appropriate combination of mitogenic and adipogenic signals to continue through the subsequent differentiation steps and the progressive acquisition of morphological and biochemical characteristics of mature adipocytes. The nature of the induction depends on the specific cell culture model used, because the responsiveness to inducing agents may vary considerably between preadipose cell lines and primary preadipocytes (6,18,35).

Generally, serum-containing medium—the standard adipogenic cocktail for induction—includes isobutylmethylxanthine (MIX), dexamethasone (DEX), and supraphysiological concentrations of insulin, abbreviated as MDI. If 3T3-L1 preadipocyte cell line cells are kept in fetal bovine serum alone, they differentiate into fat cells over several weeks. When this same cell line is immersed in DEX and MIX 48 hours after confluence, these cells begin simultaneous differentiation much earlier, roughly within five to seven days (6,18,37,38).

Following growth arrest at the G1/S cycle phase, cells that have been induced with MDI enter the cell cycle after 24 hours. They proceed to DNA replication (postconfluent mitosis) and cell doubling (clonal expansion), where transcription factors bind to the regulatory response elements in the genes that are essential for adipogenesis (18,39–41). Data collected on 3T3-L1 preadipocytes indicate that these three steps—DNA replication/synthesis, mitotic expansion, and clonal amplification—are not required steps for preadipocyte differentiation intoadipocytes (41). Thus, it has been demonstrated that pre-adipocytes that have been induced with MIX and DEX in vitro still differentiate into adipocytes without having undergone clonal expansion. Another study demonstrated that when normally induced 3T3-L1 preadipocytes are treated with a mitogen-activated protein kinase-1 (MEK-1) inhibitor, a blocker of mitotic clonal expansion through inhibition of mitogen-activated protein kinase and activation of extracellular signal-regulated kinases 1 and 2, differentiation still occurs (42–45).

Several proto-oncogenes and transcription factors aid in postconfluent mitosis and clonal expansion. The nuclear proto-oncogenes *c-fos*, *c-jun*, and *c-myc* are induced briskly—within one hour of induction with MDI to 3T3-L1 cells—and last for two to six hours thereafter. Their function is to facilitate DNA replication through cellular signaling. Transcription factors CCAAT/enhancer binding protein β (C/EBPβ) and C/EBPδ have been implicated in initiation of postconfluent mitosis and clonal expansion (44).

Following postconfluent mitosis and clonal expansion, the 3T3-L1 cell undergoes a second period of growth arrest called G_D (45). This occurs approximately two days postinduction and is a required and final step preceding terminal differentiation (45). Transcription factors peroxisome proliferator–activated receptor γ (PPARγ) and C/EBPα are key mediators of the second growth arrest that signals commitment to differentiation (45–47). At the completion of the G_D stage, preadipocytes are fully committed to differentiation. By the third day, these preadipocytes express late markers of adipocyte differentiation (8,35). By days 5 through 7, cells have completed terminal differentiation. During this time, the adipocytes have permanently withdrawn from the cell cycle, attain a spherical shape, and accumulate into fat droplets. These adipocytes also now have the ability to partake in de novo lipogenesis. This is characterized by a decrease in β1-adrenoreceptor and an increase in β2- and β3-adrenoreceptors, rendering the adipocytes more sensitive to lipolytic stimuli (48,49).

As mentioned earlier, during the final stages of terminal differentiation, the adipocyte cell shape changes from fibroblastic to spherical. This change is the prime indicator that the process of adipogenesis has begun and is accompanied by changes in the extracellular matrix (ECM) and cytoskeletal components (35). The change in the compositions of the ECM and cytoskeleton regulates adipogenesis by promoting expression of the transcription factors C/EBPα and PPARγ. For example, fibronectin, which is an important cytoskeletal component of the ECM during the initial stages of adipogenesis, inhibits adipogenesis at later stages, in part by downregulating the expression of lipogenic genes (50). During adipogenesis, the change in ECM components occurs through deposition and degradation. Matrix metalloproteinases (MMPs), a family of zinc-dependent proteinases, and their inhibitors, the tissue inhibitors of MMPs, are important mediators (51,52).

Differentiation-Associated Molecular Events

The molecular and cellular events that occur during adipocyte differentiation have been widely studied using various cell culture models, including pre-adipocyte cell lines and primary culture of adipose-derived stromal vascular precursor cells. As mentioned earlier, terminal differentiation is characterized by a permanent withdrawal of cells from the cell cycle. Genes associated with this stage are those involved in glucose and lipid metabolism, as well as production levels of the associated mRNAs, and proteins increase 10- to 100-fold.

Terminal differentiation is additionally controlled by products that are synthesized and secreted by the adipocyte itself. Its differentiation is a carefully synchronized and complex process involving coordination of multiple signals, which culminates in the expression of differentiation-dependent downstream genes, which are specific to adipocytes. For example, the expression of collagen type VI, an early marker of differentiation, and the disappearance of pref-1 (preadipocyte factor-1), an inhibitory protein, during the transition from prolif-eration to differentiation highlight just how intricate and coordinated this process is (6,18,35).

The events that take place during preadipocyte differentiation occur at the gene expression level. The elucidation of the molecular events that occur has allowed differentially regulated genes to be classified as early, intermediate, and late mRNA/protein markers. However, the pattern of gene expression is variable depending on the cell culture or protocol used in different studies (6–8,53–55). Studies using microarray technology have identified over 2000 genes (6,56).

Differentiation-Associated Transcription Factors and Signaling Molecules

PPARγ2 and the C/EBP transcription factors are important regulators of adi-pogenesis and have been the subject of intense investigation. These transcription factors are responsible for transactivation of numerous adipocyte-specific genes. After exposure to certain adipogenic induction factors, confluent preadipocytes express C/EBPβ and C/EBPδ, which in turn activate PPARγ2 and C/EBPα. The differentiating preadipocyte next produces a ligand for PPARγ2, which is the rate-limiting step. The specifics of this ligand are still unknown. Subsequently, the majority of genes that encompass the adipocyte phenotype are expressed, followed by fat accumulation. Although the process of differentiation from a nascent preadipocyte to a mature adipocyte has been widely studied and somewhat elucidated, there are details which are still unclear. A prime example is the function and transcriptional targets of the transcription factors PPARs, which are not known (6,7,54,57).

Other transcription factors that are pivotal in terminal differentiation are GATA-binding transcription factors GATA-2 and GATA-3, and cAMP response element binding protein (CREB). Expression of GATA-2 and GATA-3 inhibits adipocyte differentiation, thereby arresting cells at the preadipocyte stage.

Therefore, during differentiation, their mRNAs are downregulated, which is partly mediated through suppression of the PPARγ2 promoter. Studies have shown that embryonic stem cells that are deficient in GATA-3 are better able to differentiate into adipocytes and that GATA-2 and GATA-3 are markedly downregulated in adipose tissue of genetically obese mice (6,58,59).

CREB is another transcription factor that is crucial to adipocyte differentiation. Although it is expressed consistently before and during adipogenesis, its overexpression is enough to initiate adipogenesis. It is commonly upregulated by agents including insulin, DEX, and dibutyryl cAMP. However, in studies of cells lacking CREB, no adipogenesis occurs, even in cells treated with conventional inducing agents (6).

In addition to transcription factors, other signaling molecules such as pref-1 and Wnt also regulate adipocyte differentiation. Pref-1 is an inhibitor of adipocyte differentiation and is synthesized as a plasma membrane protein containing six epidermal growth factor (EGF)–like repeats in the extracellular domain. Pref-1 is highly expressed in 3T3-L1 preadipocytes, but is absent in mature fat cells. During adipogenesis it is downregulated, and its constitutive expression actually inhibits adipogenesis. Certain inducers, like DEX, inhibit pref-1 transcription, which, in turn, activates adipogenesis (60,61).

A signaling molecule, Wnt, like pref-1, regulates adipocyte differentiation. Studies have shown that expression of Wnt-1 or activation of its signaling cascade downstream of its receptor inhibits differentiation through the inhibition of C/EBPα and PPARγ, even when preadipocytes are treated with induction agents. Studies in 3T3-L1 preadipocytes, C3H10T1/2 cells, and NIH-3T3 fibroblasts have demonstrated that adipogenesis is activated in cell lines that have a knockout mutation of Wnt, thereby blocking its signaling cascade. Wnt also affects cell fate of mesodermal cells, as suggested by studies that showed in vitro differentiation of myoblasts into adipocytes when the Wnt pathway is inhibited (6).

CONCLUSIONS

We are just beginning to understand the complex role of adipocyte and its modulatory factors. Rapidly advancing cellular and molecular methodologies should allow us to further elucidate the myriad of functions encompassed by this intriguing cell (62).

REFERENCES

1. Burkitt HG, Young B, Heath JW. Supporting/connective tissues. In: Wheater's Functional Histology, A Text and Colour Atlas. 3rd ed. New York, NY: Churchill Livingstone, 1993:61–75.
2. Johnson PR, Greenwood MRC. The adipose tissue. In: Cell and Tissue Biology: A Textbook of Histology. 6th ed. Baltimore, MD: Urban and Schwarzenberg, 1988:191–209.

3. Brooks JSJ, Perosio PM. Adipose Tissue. In: Histology for Pathologists. 2nd ed. New York, NY: Lippincott Williams & Wilkins, 1997:167–196.
4. Klein J, Permana PA, Owecki M, et al. What are subcutaneous adipocytes really good for? Exp Dermatol 2007; 16(1):45–70.
5. MacDougald OA, Mandrup S. Adipogenesis: forces that tip the scales. Trends Endocrinol Metab 2002; 13(1):5–11.
6. Gregoire FM. Adipocyte differentiation: from fibroblast to endocrine cell. Exp Biol Med 2001; 226(11):997–1002.
7. Rosen ED, Spiegelman BM. Molecular regulation of adipogenesis. Annu Rev Cell Dev Biol 2000; 16:145–171.
8. Ntambi JM, Kim Y-C. Adipocyte differentiation and gene expression. J Nutr 2000; 130(suppl):S3122–S3126.
9. Greenwood MRC, Johnson PR. Genetic differences in adipose tissue metabolism and regulation. Ann NY Acad Sci 1993; 676:253–269.
10. Trujillo ME, Scherer PE. Adipose-derived factors: impact on health and disease. Endocr Rev 2006; 27:762–778.
11. O'Rahilly S. Human obesity and insulin resistance: lessons from experiments of human nature. Novartis Found Symp 2007; 286:13–20.
12. Patrick CW Jr. Adipose tissue engineering: the future of breast and soft tissue reconstruction following tumor resection. Semin Surg Oncol 2000; 19:302–311.
13. Katz AJ, Llull R, Hedrick MH, et al. Emerging approaches to the tissue engineering of fat. Clin Plast Surg 1999; 26:587–602.
14. Kral JG, Crandall DL. Development of a human adipocyte synthetic polymer scaffold. Plast Reconstr Surg 1999; 104:1732–1738.
15. Klein S, Coppack SW, Mohamed-Ali V, et al. Adipose tissue leptin production and plasma leptin kinetics in humans. Diabetes 1996; 45:984–987.
16. Smas CM, Sul HS. Control of adipocyte differentiation. Biochem J 1995; 309(pt 3):697–710.
17. Roche AF. The adipocyte-number hypothesis. Child Dev 1981; 52:31–43.
18. Avram MA, Avram AS, James WD. Subcutaneous fat in normal and diseased states. Adipogenesis from stem cell to fat cell. J Am Acad Dermatol 2007; 56:472–492.
19. Napolitano L. The differentiation of white adipose cells: an electron microscope study. J Cell Biol 1963; 18:663–679.
20. Pittenger MF, Mackay AM, Beck SC, et al. Multilineage potential of adult human mesenchymal stem cells. Science 1999; 284:143–147.
21. Janderova L, McNeil M, Murrell AN, et al. Human mesenchymal stem cells as an *in vitro* model for human adipogenesis. Obes Res 2003; 11:65–74.
22. Armani A, Mammi C, Marzolla V, et al. Cellular models for understanding adipogenesis, adipose dysfunction, and obesity. J Cell Biochem 2010; 110:564–572.
23. Fleishman JS, Schwartz RA. Hibernoma. Ultrastructural observations. J Surg Oncol 1983; 23:285–289.
24. Chu DH. Development and structure of skin. In: Wolff K, Goldsmith LA, Katz SI, et al. eds. Fitzpatrick's Dermatology in General Medicine. 7th ed. New York, NY: McGraw-Hill Professional, 2007.
25. Nedungadi TP, Clegg DJ. Sexual dimorphism in body fat distribution and risk for cardiovascular diseases. J Cardiovasc Trans Res 2009; 2:321–327.
26. Bjorntorp P. Body fat distribution, insulin resistance, and metabolic diseases. Nutrition 1997; 13:795–803.

27. Bays HE, Gonzalez-Campoy JM, Bray GA, et al. Pathogenic potential of adipose tissue and metabolic consequences of adipocyte hypertrophy and increased visceral adiposity. Expert Rev Cardiovasc Ther 2008; 6:343–368.
28. Green H, Kehinde O. An established preadipose cell line and its differentiation in culture. II. Factors affecting the adipose conversion. Cell 1975; 5:19–27.
29. Sugihara H, Yonemitsu N, Miyabara S, et al. Primary cultures of unilocular fat cells: characteristics of growth in vitro and changes in differentiation properties. Differentiation 1986; 31:42–49.
30. Kirkland JL, Hollenberg CH, Gillon WS. Effects of fat depot site on differentiation dependent gene expression in rat preadipocytes. Int J Obes Relat Metab Disord 1996; 20(suppl):S102–S107.
31. Hauner H, Entenmann G. Regional variation of adipose differentiation in cultured stromal-vascular cells from the abdominal and femoral adipose tissue of obese women. Int J Obes Relat Metab Disord 1991; 15:121–126.
32. Adams M, Montague CT, Prins JB, et al. Activators of PPARγ have depot-specific effects on human preadipocyte differentiation. J Clin Invest 1997; 100:3149–3153.
33. Burdi AR, Poissonnet CM, Garn SM, et al. Adipose tissue growth patterns during human gestation: a histometric comparison of buccal and gluteal fat depots. Int J Obesity Relat Metab Disord 1985; 9:247–256.
34. Prins JB, O'Rahilly S. Regulation of adipose cell number in man. Clin Sci 1997; 92:3–11.
35. Gregoire FM, Smas CM, Sul, HS. Understanding adipocyte differentiation. Physiol Rev 1998; 78:783–809.
36. Pairault J, Green H. A study of the adipose conversion of suspended 3T3 cells by using glycerophosphate dehydrogenase as differentiation marker. Proc Natl Acad Sci U S A 1979; 76:5138–5142.
37. Rubin CS, Hirsch A, Fung C, et al. Development of hormone receptors and hormonal responsiveness in vitro: Insulin receptors and insulin sensitivity in the preadipocyte and adipocyte forms of 3T3-L1 cells. J Biol Chem 1978; 253:7570–7578.
38. Green H, Kehinde O. Spontaneous heritable changes leading to increased adipose conversion in 3T3 cells. Cell 1976; 7:105–113.
39. Cornelius P, Macdougald OA, Lane MD. Regulation of adipocyte development. Annu Rev Nutr 1994; 14:99–129.
40. Bernlohr DA, Bolanowski MA, Kelly TJ, et al. Evidence for an increase in transcription of specific mRNAs during differentiation of 3T3-L1 preadipocytes. J Biol Chem 1985; 260:5563–5567.
41. Tang QQ, Otto TC, Lane MD. Mitotic clonal expansion: a synchronous process required for adipogenesis. Proc Natl Acad Sci U S A 2003; 100:44–49.
42. Qiu Z, Wei Y, Chen N, et al. DNA synthesis and mitotic clonal expansion is not a required step for 3T3-L1 preadipocytes differentiation into adipocytes. J Biol Chem 2001; 276:11988–11995.
43. Bost F, Aouadi M, Caron L, et al. The role of MAPKs in adipocyte differentiation and obesity. Biochimie 2005; 87:51–56.
44. Zhang J-W, Klemm DJ, Vinson C, et al. Role of CREB in transcriptional regulation of CCAAT/enhancer-binding protein beta gene during adipogenesis. J Biol Chem 2004; 279:4471–4478.

45. Scott RE, Florine DL, Wille JJ, et al. Coupling of growth arrest and differentiation at a distinct state in the G_1 phase of the cell cycle: G_D. Proc Natl Acad Sci U S A 1982; 79:845–849.

46. Altiok S, Xu M, Spiegelman BM. PPARγ induces cell cycle withdrawal: inhibition of E2F/DP DNA-Binding activity via down-regulation of PP2A. Genes Dev 1997; 11:1987–1998.

47. Umek RM, Friedman AD, McKnight SL. CCAAT-enhancer binding protein: a component of a differentiation switch. Science 1991; 251:288–292.

48. Guest SJ, Hadcock JR, Watkins DC, et al. β_1 and β_2 adrenergic receptor expression in differentiating 3T3-L1 cells. Independent regulation at the level of mRNA. J Biol Chem 1990; 265:5370–5375.

49. Feve B, Emorine LJ, Briend-Sutren MM, et al. Differential regulation of α_1 and β_2 adrenergic receptor protein and mRNA levels by glucocorticoids during 3T3-F442A adipose differentiation. J Biol Chem 1990; 265:16343–16349.

50. Spiegelman BM, Ginty CA. Fibronectin modulation of cell shape and lipogenic gene expression in 3T3-L1 preadipocyte differentiation. Cell 1982; 29:53–60.

51. Vu TH, Werb Z. Matrix metalloproteinases: effectors of development and normal physiology. Genes Dev 2000; 14:2123–2133.

52. Chavey C, Mari B, Monthouel M-N, et al. Matrix metalloproteinases are differentially expressed in adipose tissue during obesity and modulate adipocyte differentiation. J Biol Chem 2003; 278:11888–11896.

53. Morrison RF, Farmer SR. Hormonal signaling and transcriptional control of adipocyte differentiation. J Nutr 2000; 130:3116S–3121S.

54. Rangwala SM, Lazar MA. Transcriptional control of adipogenesis. Annu Rev Nutr 2000; 20:535–559.

55. Boone C, Mourot J, Gregoire F, et al. The adipose conversion process: regulation by extracellular and intracellular factors. Reprod Nutr Dev 2000; 40:325–358.

56. Guo X, Liao K. Analysis of gene expression profile during 3T3-L1 preadipocyte differentiation. Gene 2000; 251:45–53.

57. Zhao L, Gregoire F, Sul HS. Transient induction of ENC-1, a Kelch-related actin-binding protein, is required for adipocyte differentiation. J Biol Chem 2000; 275:16845–16850.

58. Reusch JE, Colton LA, Klemm DJ. CREB activation induces adipogenesis in 3T3-L1 cells. Mol Cell Biol 2000; 20:1008–1020.

59. Tong Q, Dalgin G, Xu H, et al. Function of GATA transcription factors in pre-adipocyte-adipocyte transition. Science 2000; 290:134–138.

60. Ross SE, Hemati N, Longo KA, et al. Inhibition of adipogenesis by Wnt signaling. Science 2000; 289:950–953.

61. Sul HS, Smas C, Mei B, et al. Function of pref-1 as an inhibitor of adipocyte differentiation. Int J Obes Relat Metab Disord 2000; 24(suppl 4):S15–S19.

62. Sharma PK, Janniger CK, Schwartz RA, et al. The treatment of atypical lipoma with liposuction. J Dermatol Surg Oncol 1991; 17:332–334.

2

Physiology, pathophysiology, and aging

Alexander L. Berlin

INTRODUCTION

In the previous chapter, the embryology and structure of human adipose tissue have been explored. In the current chapter, we focus on the function of the adipocytes, both in health and in disease. In addition, changes associated with physiological aging of fat will also be explored.

BACKGROUND

The classical view of the adipose tissue function is that of storage of excess energy, which could be mobilized during times of food deprivation or starvation. Additionally, subcutaneous fat protects the underlying organs, provides thermal insulation, and allows for a smoother body shape, a fact that becomes evident in conditions known as lipodystrophies. More recently, however, adipose tissue was revealed to be an active endocrine and paracrine organ that participates in the production of numerous hormones, cytokines, and other physiologically active peptides. It also actively participates in glucose and lipid metabolism and serves as a source of stem cells. It should be no wonder then that either excess fatty tissue, in the form of obesity, or its paucity, as represented by lipodystrophies, can lead to numerous systemic disorders.

CURRENT STATE OF KNOWLEDGE

Adipose tissue appears to be a very heterogeneous organ, with significant differences in cellular composition and physiological function between depots. Thus, as discussed in the previous chapter, adipose tissue is generally subdivided into white adipose tissue (WAT) and brown adipose tissue (BAT). In addition,

WAT is typically further classified as intra-abdominal versus subcutaneous in localization.

WHITE ADIPOSE TISSUE

Lipid Metabolism

Quantitatively, the most significant function of the adipocytes is the storage of lipids in the form of triacylglycerols (TGs)—also known as triglycerides—for later use as an energy substrate by the body. Although fatty acids are readily synthesized de novo from glucose in the liver, this process is very limited in the adipose tissue (1). Thus, most lipids contained within the adipocytes are derived from dietary intake and hepatic production.

The availability of free fatty acids (FFAs) for uptake into the fatty tissue is regulated by lipoprotein lipase (LPL), an adipocyte-derived enzyme. Following its synthesis and secretion, LPL is bound to the capillary wall, where it hydrolyzes fatty acids from TGs within very low-density lipoproteins (VLDLs) and chylomicrons from circulation (2). LPL synthesis and activity are upregulated by numerous factors, including high body mass index (BMI), hyperinsulinemia, hypercortisolemia, and elevated levels of peroxisome proliferator–activated receptor (PPAR)-gamma, as described below (2–8). On the other hand, its activity is downregulated by several factors, including epinephrine, growth hormone, FFAs, testosterone, tumor necrosis factor (TNF)-alpha, interferon-gamma, and leukemia inhibitory factor (9–16).

Following hydrolysis, FFAs are transported across the adipocyte cellular membrane via a fatty acid transport protein (FATP) and are subsequently bound by the cytosolic adipocyte lipid-binding protein (aP2) (17). FFAs are then esterified through the action of acyl-coenzyme A (acyl-CoA) synthetase and are bound to a backbone of glycerol—itself a product of adipocyte glucose metabolism, as discussed in section "Glucose Metabolism" below—to successively form mono , di-, and, ultimately, triacylglycerols (Fig. 2.1). The rate of TG synthesis differs between adipose tissue depots; thus, synthesis within intra-abdominal, or omental, fat is slower than that within the subcutaneous adipose tissue (18).

Recently, PPARs, a family of ligand-activated transcription factors from the nuclear hormone receptor superfamily, have also been implicated in lipid metabolism (19). Three factors, alpha, delta (also known as beta), and gamma, have been identified so far in human beings. In general, PPARs act by forming heterodimers with the retinoid X receptors (RXR) and binding to DNA response elements, thereby activating specific gene transcription. In addition to its function as a promoter of adipogenesis, as described in the previous chapter, PPAR-gamma enhances FFA uptake and TG storage by the adipocytes. This is achieved through several mechanisms, including the stimulation of LPL, FATP, intracellular FFA transport, acyl-CoA synthase, esterification of FFA to TG, and the promotion of more efficient TG storage within the lipid droplets (20,21).

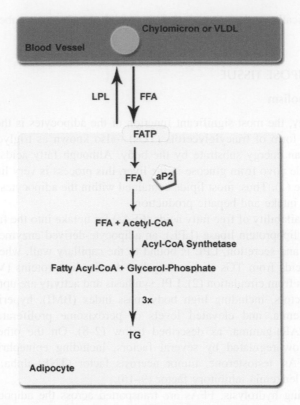

Figure 2.1 Schematic representation of human lipogenesis. *Abbreviations*: aP2, adipocyte lipid-binding protein; CoA, coenzyme A; FATP, fatty acid transport protein; FFA, free fatty acid; LPL, lipoprotein lipase; TG, triacylglycerol; VLDL, very low density lipoprotein.

Additionally, PPAR-gamma directly affects the synthesis of cellular adipokines, such as adiponectin, described in section "Endocrine Functions" below (22). PPAR-delta and PPAR-alpha may further contribute to lipid metabolism through the upregulation of FFA oxidation and the increased expression of uncoupling protein, UCP-1, as presented in section "Brown Adipose Tissue" below (23–25).

    On the other end of adipose tissue lipid metabolism is lipolysis, the process of hydrolysis of TGs to FFA and glycerol for subsequent release into the bloodstream and utilization by other peripheral organs through beta-oxidation or re-esterification by the adipocytes. This process ensures an adequate energy supply to peripheral tissues during fasting or increased energy requirements. Lipolysis is regulated by hormone-sensitive lipase (HSL), which hydrolyzes TGs

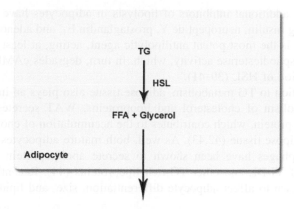

Figure 2.2 Schematic representation of human lipolysis. *Abbreviations*: FFA, free fatty acid; HSL, hormone-sensitive lipase; TG, triacylglycerol.

into diacylglycerol and monoacylglycerol (Fig. 2.2). Although additional regulatory mechanisms have been proposed (26), the enzyme is primarily activated through phosphorylation by cAMP-dependent protein kinase A (27–29). The main regulators of lipolysis in human adipocytes are catecholamines—epinephrine and norepinephrine (30), with additional limited stimulation by the growth hormone (31).

Human adipocytes possess both agonistic (beta-1, -2, and -3) and antagonistic (alpha-2) adrenergic receptors (30,32–35). The agonistic adrenoceptors interact with stimulatory G (G_s) proteins, which activate adenylate cyclase, the enzyme responsible for cyclic adenosine monophosphate (cAMP) production. As described above, this results in the activation of HSL and subsequent increased lipolysis. Alternatively, antagonistic adrenoceptors interact with inhibitory G (G_i) proteins and inhibit adenylate cyclase, leading to the dephosphorylation of HSL and decreased lipolysis.

It appears that there are regional and gender variations in the distribution of both beta and alpha-2 adrenoceptors (36,37), which may lead to differential responses to catecholamines and account, at least in part, for variations in the sites of fat deposition. For example, lipolysis in response to catecholamines was found to be significantly higher in abdominal subcutaneous adipose tissue as compared to gluteal fat depots, which was more prominent in females. This corresponded to a much higher beta-adrenergic sensitivity and much lower alpha-adrenergic sensitivity in the abdominal versus gluteal adipocytes (37). As well, visceral adipose tissue in severely obese female patients demonstrated decreased alpha adrenoceptor sensitivity and, subsequently, a higher rate of lipolysis as compared to abdominal subcutaneous adipocytes (38).

Several additional inhibitors of lipolysis in adipocytes have been identified, including insulin, neuropeptide Y, prostaglandin E_1, and adenosine (34). Of these, insulin is the most potent antilipolytic agent, acting, at least partially, by inducing phosphodiesterase activity, which, in turn, degrades cAMP and results in the inhibition of HSL (39–41).

In addition to TG metabolism, adipose tissue also plays an important role in the metabolism of cholesterol and lipoproteins. WAT secretes cholesteryl ester transfer protein, which contributes to the accumulation of cholesteryl ester within the adipose tissue (42,43). As well, both mature adipocytes and adipose tissue macrophages have been shown to secrete apolipoprotein E (apoE), a component of VLDL and other TG-rich lipoproteins (44). Recently, apoE has also been shown to affect adipocyte differentiation, size, and lipid metabolism (45).

Glucose Metabolism

In addition to lipid metabolism, adipose tissue actively participates in glucose metabolism. Glucose transporter (GLUT) proteins, mostly GLUT4 and, to a lesser extent, GLUT1, transport glucose into the cytosol of the adipocytes (46). GLUT4 activity is highly dependent on insulin (47,48) and its expression has been found to be significantly reduced in obese individuals, thus contributing to insulin resistance (49).

Once inside the cytosol, the glucose molecule can follow one of several distinct metabolic pathways. It has been estimated that over 50% of the oral glucose load may be metabolized to lactate within the adipose tissue of obese individuals (50). Lactate is then secreted into the bloodstream and may be used for hepatic gluconeogenesis or glycogen synthesis, depending on the nutritional status. Alternatively, glucose may be converted to glycerol and become incorporated into TGs, broken down to CO_2 moieties, or utilized in the de novo synthesis of FFA. The latter pathway and two enzymes associated with it—acetyl-CoA carboxylase and fatty acid synthase—have been extensively studied because of their potential contribution to the pathogenesis of obesity (51,52).

In addition to these processes within the fat cells, FFAs and several adipokines secreted by the adipose tissue affect glucose uptake and metabolism within other peripheral organs, including muscle cells and the liver, and thus contribute to increased gluconeogenesis and insulin resistance (53–55).

Endocrine Functions

The concept of adipose tissue as an endocrine organ is quite recent and new discoveries in this field are contributing to a growing list of adipocyte-derived proteins and peptides, collectively known as adipokines (56). In this chapter, we will examine some of the best studied of these molecules, including leptin, adiponectin, resistin, and TNF-alpha.

Leptin—from the Greek word "leptos" meaning thin—was the first adipokine to be discovered (57). Most synthesis occurs within the WAT, with subcutaneous tissue expressing higher levels of this protein as compared to intra-abdominal fat (58). Leptin appears to signal adequate energy storage to the brain so that its levels are low during starvation and high in obese individuals (59). Leptin receptors have been found in most tissues, thus accounting for the numerous functions of this hormone (60). In the hypothalamus, leptin causes the upregulation and release of anorexigenic neurotransmitters, such as neuropeptide Y, thereby decreasing oral food intake (61). Peripherally, leptin increases insulin sensitivity, reduces insulin secretion by the pancreas, increases lipolysis and fatty acid oxidation, and decreases lipogenesis (62–65). Furthermore, leptin has been found to increase platelet aggregation, promote angiogenesis, and affect the immune system, including T-cells, monocytes, and endothelial adhesion molecules (66–71). Leptin from subcutaneous adipocytes has also been shown to be an important factor in cutaneous wound healing, acting on keratinocytes, fibroblasts, and cutaneous vasculature (72).

Adiponectin is a protein with homology to collagen that is synthesized and secreted by the adipocytes. As opposed to that of most other adipokines, plasma levels of adiponectin are high in lean individuals and fall in obese, insulin-resistant, or diabetic patients (73,74). Adiponectin improves peripheral insulin resistance through increased fatty acid oxidation, increased glucose uptake, and decreased hepatic gluconeogenesis (75,76). Adiponectin also appears to have anti-atherogenic properties, including decreased monocyte adhesion to endothelial cells and reduced transformation of macrophages into foam cells (77–80). Thus, reduced levels of adiponectin may serve as a link between obesity and atherosclerosis. Finally, adiponectin appears to have anti-inflammatory properties, inhibiting the production of TNF-alpha and upregulating the synthesis of IL-10 and IL-1 receptor antagonists (81–83).

Resistin was originally proposed to be a possible molecular link between obesity and diabetes. In murine models, resistin levels were elevated in obesity, recombinant resistin increased peripheral insulin resistance and hepatic gluconeogenesis, and antibodies to resistin improved insulin sensitivity and decreased serum glucose (54,84). Murine resistin was found to be almost exclusively expressed by adipocytes (54). In contrast, human adipose tissue is a relatively minor contributor to the production of resistin, with stromal monocytes and macrophages—rather than the adipocytes—synthesizing this polypeptide (85,86). Increased resistin levels have been found in many inflammatory processes such as coronary atherosclerosis (87–89), endothelial dysfunction (90,91), connective tissue diseases including rheumatoid arthritis and systemic lupus erythematosus (92–94), psoriasis (95), and inflammatory bowel diseases (96); however, its specific role in these diseases has yet to be elucidated and confirmed in future studies.

TNF-alpha is a "classic" cytokine also synthesized and secreted by macrophages within the adipose tissue (97). Originally, TNF-alpha was also proposed to be the molecular link between obesity and insulin resistance (98,99). Studies have demonstrated the induction of insulin resistance in TNF-alpha–exposed animals and the reversal of this effect following treatment with a soluble TNF-alpha receptor (100). Within the adipose tissue, TNF-alpha induces lipolysis and suppresses lipogenesis (101,102). On the other hand, the cytokine stimulates fatty acid synthesis and decreases fatty acid oxidation in the liver (103). The overall effect is that of hypertriglyceridemia. In addition, TNF-alpha inactivates the insulin receptor and insulin receptor substrate 1 and reduces the synthesis of adiponectin by the adipocytes in a paracrine manner (104,105). However, it is unclear whether adipose tissue production of TNF-alpha directly contributes to its serum concentration in obese individuals. As well, TNF-alpha neutralization did not improve insulin sensitivity in a study of obese diabetic patients (106). Instead, the cytokine was found to increase the production of various factors that may contribute to inflammation and cardiovascular disease, such as transforming growth factor (TGF)-beta, plasminogen activator inhibitor-1, IL-6, and monocyte chemoattractant protein (MCP)-1 (105,107,108).

Clearly, the function of WAT goes far beyond the simple storage of nutrients for later utilization during the times of fasting. Instead, it is a complex tissue, which affects most organs in the human body. Future studies will likely reveal new and important information about the physiology of adipocytes.

BROWN ADIPOSE TISSUE

Long thought to be mainly limited to lower animals and neonates, BAT appears to also play an important physiological role in human adults. As discussed in the previous chapter, in adults, brown fat is mainly present under the skin of the back and shoulders. In addition, it has been estimated that approximately 1 in 100 to 200 intraperitoneal fat cells within WAT is actually a brown adipocyte (109).

The main function of brown fat appears to be the conversion of food into energy in the form of heat. To that effect, brown adipocytes express a unique mitochondrial protein UCP-1, also known as thermogenin (110). In BAT, as in most other tissues, electron donor molecules, such as NADH, generated from fatty acid or glucose metabolism transfer their electrons down the electron transport chain to an electron acceptor—typically the oxygen molecule. In the process, protons are pumped out of the mitochondrial matrix and into the intermembrane space. This creates a pH and an electrochemical gradient across the inner mitochondrial membrane. In most tissues, the gradient is then coupled to oxidative phosphorylation, a process of conversion of adenosine diphosphate (ADP) to adenosine triphosphate (ATP) by ATP synthase. In brown fat, however, UCP-1, an inner mitochondrial wall protein, allows the leakage of protons back into the mitochondrial matrix, thus uncoupling the electron transport chain from the process of oxidative phosphorylation. As a result, the

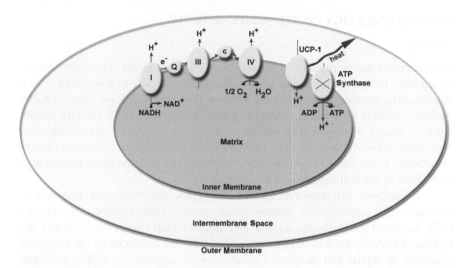

Figure 2.3 Electron transport chain in the mitochondrion of a brown adipocyte. *Abbreviations*: I, complex I; III, complex III; IV, complex IV; ADP, adenosine diphosphate; ATP, adenosine triphosphate; c, cytochrome *c*; e$^-$, electron; NADH, nicotinamide adenine dinucleotide; Q, coenzyme Q; UCP-1, uncoupling protein 1. *Source*: From Ref. 111.

energy generated by the electron transport chain is released in the form of heat (Fig. 2.3) (111).

UCP-1 appears to be uniquely responsible for the process of adaptive nonshivering thermogenesis, which accounts for acclimation in response to prolonged cold exposure and for heat production during the postnatal period and febrile illnesses (112–114). The process is mainly regulated by the sympathetic nervous system through beta-3 adrenergic receptors expressed in brown adipocytes (115).

There is evidence to suggest that, because of decreased metabolic efficiency of food associated with the activation of UCP-1, BAT may impart protection against obesity. In murine studies, ablation or inactivation of brown fat has resulted in lowered body temperature and obese, insulin-resistant specimens (116,117). In humans, various polymorphisms in the beta-3 adrenoceptor and UCP-1 have been shown to be associated with a greater propensity toward obesity in several studies (118–120). However, this correlation has not yet been firmly confirmed; as well, further work is needed to delineate the precise function of the more recently discovered uncoupling proteins, especially UCP-2 and UCP-3 (121). Nonetheless, the activation of brown adipocytes may represent a viable future therapeutic option in the treatment of obesity (122).

PATHOPHYSIOLOGY OF THE ADIPOSE TISSUE

Obesity

It is estimated that nearly a third of adults in the United States is currently obese, as are over 17% of children and adolescents (123). Obesity is associated with a significantly increased incidence of various chronic conditions, most notably diabetes mellitus type 2 and cardiovascular diseases (124,125). Obesity results from an excess dietary energy intake, a deficiency of energy expenditure, or, frequently, a combination thereof. In addition, as discussed previously in section "Endocrine Functions", various genetic mutations and inflammatory factors also contribute to the pathogenesis of this condition.

It has been demonstrated that as adipocytes hypertrophy in response to excessive food consumption, adipose tissue becomes infiltrated by macrophages (97). Activated macrophages release TNF-alpha, which causes lipolysis and the release of FFAs by the adipocytes (126). This is further enhanced by the enhanced synthesis of leptin and decreased production of adiponectin within enlarged adipocytes. FFAs then directly activate macrophages through Toll-like receptor (TLR)-4, leading to an even greater production of TNF-alpha (127). In addition to this mutual paracrine activation by the adipocytes and the macrophages, TNF-alpha also leads to the synthesis and release of other proinflammatory factors, such as IL-6, intracellular adhesion molecule (ICAM)-1, and MCP-1, which lead to further influx of monocytes and their differentiation into tissue macrophages (105). This establishes a chronic low-grade inflammatory state, believed to be an important contributor to the pathophysiology of obesity.

Like a vicious cycle, obesity, in turn, leads to the dysfunction of adipose tissue. Thus, obese individuals demonstrate high levels of leptin but poor appetite control. This has led to the concept of leptin resistance (128). Leptin resistance also contributes to insulin resistance, likewise leading to abnormal regulation of food intake and body weight (129).

It should become clear from the above discussion that obesity is a multifactorial, polygenic disorder, so that a successful, long-term treatment may require multiple coordinated therapeutic approaches.

Lipodystrophies

On the other end of the spectrum of pathophysiological conditions affecting the adipose tissue are lipodystrophies. A heterogeneous group of conditions, lipodystrophies are characterized by generalized or localized loss of adipocytes, sometimes associated with a compensatory lipohypertrophy in unaffected sites. Lipodystrophies are also frequently associated with significant metabolic disturbances.

Lipodystrophies are typically divided into congenital/familial and acquired, and are further subdivided into generalized, partial, and localized. In addition to various systemic manifestations, most lipodystrophies, including congenital generalized lipodystrophy (Berardinelli–Seip syndrome), familial partial lipodystrophy (Kobberling–Dunnigan syndrome), acquired generalized lipodystrophy (Lawrence syndrome), and HIV-related lipodystrophy linked to highly active antiretroviral therapy (HAART)—see below—are associated with moderate to pronounced insulin resistance, diabetes mellitus type 2, and hypertriglyceridemia (130). These conditions illustrate well the crucial importance of functional adipose tissue to the metabolic equilibrium and to the overall health of the individual.

This chapter examines the most common lipodystrophy encountered in clinical practice today, that of HIV/HAART-associated lipodystrophy syndrome (HAART-LDS). For more information on the other congenital and acquired lipodystrophies, the reader is invited to review recent articles on the subject (130,131).

First reported in 1998, the HAART-LDS has been described with the use of protease inhibitors (PIs) and nucleoside reverse transcriptase inhibitors (NRTIs) and is thought to occur in approximately 50% or more of HIV-infected patients treated with these medications (132–134). Clinically, lipoatrophy of the face, limbs, and buttocks may be noted, as may lipohypertrophy of the dorso-cervical fat pad (also known as "buffalo hump"), abdomen, and breasts, or a combination thereof. In the face, the most prominent features are typically the loss of buccal and temporal fat pads, with subsequent preauricular and cheek concavities, as well as periorbital hollowing and prominent nasolabial folds (135). Additionally, hypercholesterolemia, hypertriglyceridemia, insulin resistance, and diabetes mellitus type 2 are also frequently observed in conjunction with this syndrome (133,136). Histologically, lipoatrophic adipose tissue in the HAART-LDS is characterized by a reduced adipocyte size, decreased adipogenesis, macrophage infiltration, and fibrosis (137). Moreover, adipocyte apoptosis has also been demonstrated (138).

Although the exact pathophysiological mechanism underlying the etiology of the HAART-LDS has not been fully elucidated, several hypotheses have been proposed. PIs may target two human proteins partially homologous with HIV protease: cytoplasmic retinoic acid–binding protein (CRABP)-1, which normally forms a heterodimer with PPAR-gamma and inhibits adipocyte apoptosis while enhancing preadipocyte differentiation, and LDL receptor–related protein, an essential component of the hepatic chylomicron uptake and endothelial TG clearance (139). PI-mediated impairment in the nuclear localization of sterol regulatory element–binding protein (SREBP)-1 has been suggested to further contribute to decreased adipocyte differentiation, increased apoptosis, and insulin resistance (140). There is also evidence that some NRTIs may lead to mitochondrial toxicity and subsequent adipocyte apoptosis (141,142). Finally, an altered expression of adipokines, most notably an increased expression of proinflammatory, proapoptotic TNF-alpha and IL-6, as well as that of the monocyte chemokine MCP-1, accompanied by a decreased secretion of anti-inflammatory, insulin-sensitizing adiponectin, has also been observed in adipocytes exposed to both PIs and NRTIs (137,143–145). These findings appear to be in agreement with the above-noted macrophage infiltration into the adipose tissue in lipodystrophic areas, thus suggesting a likely important role of low-grade inflammation in the pathogenesis of the HAART-LDS.

Much more than a cosmetic concern, both the excess and paucity of adipose tissue are associated with significant metabolic, endocrine, and systemic organ dysfunction, and, consequently, significant morbidity and mortality.

AGING OF THE ADIPOSE TISSUE

As the adipose tissue ages, numerous physiological changes take place, resulting in the redistribution of fat depots with prominent anatomical transformation. Most notably, an increase in the amount of visceral adipose tissue and fat content in nonadipose tissues, such as the bone marrow, muscle, and myocardium, has been noted, together with accompanying lipoatrophy of subcutaneous fat, including that of the face (146–149). Such redistribution has important implications for morbidity and mortality, including higher risk of dyslipidemia, coronary artery disease, and insulin resistance (150,151).

Although the number of preadipocytes increases in many fat depots with aging, their ability to form mature adipocytes through the process of adipogenesis, as well as their capacity to accumulate lipids, is diminished, leading to a decreased adipocyte size (152–155). Adipogenesis appears to be influenced by the age-associated decrease in proadipogenic transcription factors, such as CCAAT/enhancer binding protein (C/EBP)-alpha (156) and steroid receptor coactivator (SRC)-1 (with subsequent reduced PPAR-gamma activity) (157), as well as by a concomitant increase in anti-adipogenic regulators, such as CUG triplet repeat-binding protein (CUGBP1) (158), C/EBP-beta liver inhibitory protein (156), C/EBP homologous protein (CHOP), and TNF-alpha (159). The exact mechanisms for the difference in fat mass accretion versus loss in various depots have not yet been elucidated, but may be related to depot-specific variations in the expression of these or other factors (160).

In addition to the process of adipogenesis, the above-mentioned adipokines and cellular factors may also affect glucose and lipid metabolism, thus leading to age-associated changes in the physiology of the adipose tissue. For example, reduced expression of C/EBP-alpha negatively affects the expression of GLUT4 and, therefore, contributes to impaired glucose tolerance (161). Likewise, age-associated decreased levels of the aP2—essential for FFA uptake—may be related to reduced C/EBP-alpha and PPAR-gamma activities (162). Furthermore, age-associated increased TNF-alpha expression by the adipose tissue may contribute to depot-specific lipolysis and smaller adipocyte size; however, its direct contribution to insulin resistance is debatable (101,104,159,163).

In the facial region, age-associated lipoatrophy is best analyzed in terms of separate anatomical regions, with the periorbital, temple, and mid-face regions being most commonly affected. Thus, in the periorbital area, infraorbital hollowing along the orbital rim results in the so-called "tear trough" deformity; however, the orbital rim is also exaggerated superiorly and laterally and contributes to the apparent redundancy in the upper eyelid skin (148). Age-related atrophy of the temporal fat pads contributes to the concavity of the temples, mid-facial descent, and prominence of the zygomatic arch (148). Deep mid-facial fat may be the most important determinant of mid-face and cheek aging as volume loss in this area may lead to a diminished support for the medial cheek compartment and subsequent nasolabial fold descent and jowl protrusion (164).

Not surprisingly, the knowledge of physiological and anatomical changes associated with aging is of utmost importance to the various treatment modalities, as described in subsequent chapters.

CONCLUSIONS

The intricate details of adipose tissue physiology only recently began to be uncovered, leading to a new understanding of the importance of this organ to the health of the entire organism. Such understanding will undoubtedly lead to new developments in the treatment of diseases associated with pathological conditions of fat. Perhaps most importantly, a greater appreciation of the various factors involved in the aging of the adipose tissue may, at some point, allow their reversal with subsequent increase in human longevity.

REFERENCES

1. Angel A, Bray GA. Synthesis of fatty acids and cholesterol by liver, adipose tissue and intestinal mucosa from obese and control patients. Eur J Clin Invest 1979; 9(5):355–362.
2. Eckel RH. Lipoprotein lipase. A multifunctional enzyme relevant to common metabolic diseases. N Engl J Med 1989; 320(16):1060–1068.
3. Ong JM, Kern PA. Effect of feeding and obesity on lipoprotein lipase activity, immunoreactive protein, and messenger RNA levels in human adipose tissue. J Clin Invest 1989; 84(1):305–311.
4. Pykalisto OJ, Smith PH, Brunzell JD. Determinants of human adipose tissue lipoprotein lipase. Effect of diabetes and obesity on basal- and diet-induced activity. J Clin Invest 1975; 56(5):1108–1117.
5. Sadur CN, Eckel RH. Insulin stimulation of adipose tissue lipoprotein lipase. Use of the euglycemic clamp technique. J Clin Invest 1982; 69(5):1119–1125.
6. Appel B, Fried SK. Effects of insulin and dexamethasone on lipoprotein lipase in human adipose tissue. Am J Physiol 1992; 262(5 pt 1):E695–E699.
7. Rebuffe-Scrive M, Krotkiewski M, Elfverson J, et al. Muscle and adipose tissue morphology and metabolism in Cushing's syndrome. J Clin Endocrinol Metab 1988; 67(6):1122–1128.
8. Cigolini M, Smith U. Human adipose tissue in culture. VIII. Studies on the insulin-antagonistic effect of glucocorticoids. Metabolism 1979; 28(5):502–510.

9. Ashby P, Robinson DS. Effects of insulin, glucocorticoids, and adrenaline on the activity of rat adipose tissue lipoprotein lipase. Biochem J 1980; 188(1):185–192.

10. Ball KL, Speake BK, Robinson DS. Effects of adrenaline on the turnover of lipoprotein lipase in rat adipose tissue. Biochim Biophys Acta 1986; 877(3):399–405.

11. Asayama K, Amemiya S, Kusano S, et al. Growth-hormone-induced changes in postheparin plasma lipoprotein lipase and hepatic triglyceride lipase activities. Metabolism 1984; 33(2):129–131.

12. Richelsen B, Pedersen SB, Borglum JD, et al. Growth hormone treatment of obese women for 5 wk: effect on body composition and adipose tissue LPL activity. Am J Physiol 1994; 266(2 pt 1):E211–E216.

13. Marin P, Oden B, Bjorntorp P. Assimilation and mobilization of triglycerides in subcutaneous abdominal and femoral adipose tissue in vivo in men: effects of androgens. J Clin Endocrinol Metab 1995; 80(1):239–243.

14. Kern PA, Saghizadeh M, Ong JM, et al. The expression of tumor necrosis factor in human adipose tissue. Regulation by obesity, weight loss, and relationship to lipoprotein lipase. J Clin Invest 1995; 95(5):2111–2119.

15. Hardardottir I, Doerrler W, Feingold KR, et al. Cytokines stimulate lipolysis and decrease lipoprotein lipase activity in cultured fat cells by a prostaglandin independent mechanism. Biochem Biophys Res Commun 1992; 186(1):237–243.

16. Marshall MK, Doerrler W, Feingold KR, et al. Leukemia inhibitory factor induces changes in lipid metabolism in cultured adipocytes. Endocrinology 1994; 135(1): 141–147.

17. Stahl A, Gimeno RE, Tartaglia LA, et al. Fatty acid transport proteins: a current view of a growing family. Trends Endocrinol Metab 2001; 12(6):266–273.

18. Maslowska MH, Sniderman AD, MacLean LD, et al. Regional differences in triacylglycerol synthesis in adipose tissue and in cultured preadipocytes. J Lipid Res 1993; 34(2):219–228.

19. Feige JN, Gelman L, Michalik L, et al. From molecular action to physiological outputs: peroxisome proliferator-activated receptors are nuclear receptors at the crossroads of key cellular functions. Prog Lipid Res 2006; 45(2):120–159.

20. Christodoulides C, Vidal-Puig A. PPARs and adipocyte function. Mol Cell Endocrinol 2010; 318(1–2):61–68.

21. Nishino N, Tamori Y, Tateya S, et al. FSP27 contributes to efficient energy storage in murine white adipocytes by promoting the formation of unilocular lipid droplets. J Clin Invest 2008; 118(8):2808–2821.

22. Maeda N, Takahashi M, Funahashi T, et al. PPARgamma ligands increase expression and plasma concentrations of adiponectin, an adipose-derived protein. Diabetes 2001; 50(9):2094–2099.

23. Wang YX, Lee CH, Tiep S, et al. Peroxisome-proliferator-activated receptor delta activates fat metabolism to prevent obesity. Cell 2003; 113(2):159–170.

24. Cabrero A, Alegret M, Sanchez RM, et al. Bezafibrate reduces mRNA levels of adipocyte markers and increases fatty acid oxidation in primary culture of adipocytes. Diabetes 2001; 50(8):1883–1890.

25. Xue B, Coulter A, Rim JS, et al. Transcriptional synergy and the regulation of Ucp1 during brown adipocyte induction in white fat depots. Mol Cell Biol 2005; 25(18):8311–8322.

26. Egan JJ, Greenberg AS, Chang MK, et al. Mechanism of hormone-stimulated lipolysis in adipocytes: translocation of hormone-sensitive lipase to the lipid storage droplet. Proc Natl Acad Sci U S A 1992; 89(18):8537–8541.

27. Garton AJ, Campbell DG, Cohen P, et al. Primary structure of the site on bovine hormone-sensitive lipase phosphorylated by cyclic AMP-dependent protein kinase. FEBS Lett 1988; 229(1):68–72.

28. Holm C, Belfrage P, Fredrikson G. Human adipose tissue hormone-sensitive lipase: identification and comparison with other species. Biochim Biophys Acta 1989; 1006(2):193–197.

29. Stralfors P, Bjorgell P, Belfrage P. Hormonal regulation of hormone-sensitive lipase in intact adipocytes: identification of phosphorylated sites and effects on the phosphorylation by lipolytic hormones and insulin. Proc Natl Acad Sci U S A 1984; 81(11):3317–3321.

30. Coppack SW, Jensen MD, Miles JM. In vivo regulation of lipolysis in humans. J Lipid Res 1994; 35(2):177–193.

31. Goodman H, Grichting G. Growth hormone and lipolysis: a reevaluation. Endocrinology 1983; 113(5):1697–1702.

32. Langin D, Tavernier G, Lafontan M. Regulation of beta 3-adrenoceptor expression in white fat cells. Fundam Clin Pharmacol 1995; 9(2):97–106.

33. Lonnqvist F, Thome A, Nilsell K, et al. A pathogenic role of visceral fat beta 3-adrenoceptors in obesity. J Clin Invest 1995; 95(3):1109–1116.

34. Castan I, Valet P, Quideau N, et al. Antilipolytic effects of alpha 2-adrenergic agonists, neuropeptide Y, adenosine, and PGE1 in mammal adipocytes. Am J Physiol 1994; 266(4 pt 2):R1141–R1147.

35. Berlan M, Lafontan M. Evidence that epinephrine acts preferentially as an antilipolytic agent in abdominal human subcutaneous fat cells: assessment by analysis of beta and alpha 2 adrenoceptor properties. Eur J Clin Invest 1985; 15(6):341–348.

36. Mauriege P, Galitzky J, Berlan M, et al. Heterogeneous distribution of beta and alpha-2 adrenoceptor binding sites in human fat cells from various deposits: functional consequences. Eur J Clin Invest 1987; 17(2):156–165.

37. Wahrenberg H, Lonnqvist F, Arner P. Mechanisms underlying regional differences in lipolysis in human adipose tissue. J Clin Invest 1989; 84(2):458–467.

38. Mauriege P, Marette A, Atgie C, et al. Regional variation in adipose tissue metabolism of severely obese premenopausal women. J Lipid Res 1995; 36(4):672–684.

39. Coppack SW, Frayn KN, Humphreys SM, et al. Effects of insulin on human adipose tissue metabolism in vivo. Clin Sci (Lond) 1989; 77(6):663–670.

40. Jensen MD, Caruso M, Heiling V, et al. Insulin regulation of lipolysis in nondiabetic and IDDM subjects. Diabetes 1989; 38(12):1595–1601.

41. Eriksson H, Ridderstrale M, Degerman E, et al. Evidence for the key role of the adipocyte cGMP-inhibited cAMP phosphodiesterase in the antilipolytic action of insulin. Biochim Biophys Acta 1995; 1266(1):101–107.

42. Radeau T, Lau P, Robb M, et al. Cholesteryl ester transfer protein (CETP) mRNA abundance in human adipose tissue: relationship to cell size and membrane cholesterol content. J Lipid Res 1995; 36(12):2552–2561.

43. Radeau T, Robb M, McDonnell M, et al. Preferential expression of cholesteryl ester transfer protein mRNA by stromal-vascular cells of human adipose tissue. Biochim Biophys Acta 1998; 1392(2-3):245–253.

44. Zechner R, Moser R, Newman TC, et al. Apolipoprotein E gene expression in mouse 3T3–L1 adipocytes and human adipose tissue and its regulation by differentiation. J Biol Chem 1991; 266(16):10583–10588.

45. Huang ZH, Reardon CA, Mazzone T. Endogenous ApoE expression modulates adipocyte triglyceride content and turnover. Diabetes 2006; 55(12):3394–3402.

46. Zorzano A, Wilkinson W, Kotliar N, et al. Insulin-regulated glucose uptake in rat adipocytes is mediated by two transporter isoforms present in at least vesicle populations. J Biol Chem 1989; 264(21):12358–12363.

47. Czech MP. Molecular actions of insulin on glucose transport. Annu Rev Nutr 1995; 15:441–471.

48. McGowan KM, Long SD, Pekala PH. Glucose transporter gene expression: regulation of transcription and mRNA stability. Pharmacol Ther 1995; 66(3):465–505.

49. Giacchetti G, Faloia E, Taccaliti A, et al. Decreased expression of insulin-sensitive glucose transporter mRNA (GLUT4) in adipose tissue of non-insulin-dependent diabetic and obese patients: evaluation by a simplified quantitative PCR assay. J Endocrinol Invest 1994; 17(9):709–715.

50. Digirolamo M, Newby FD, Lovejoy J. Lactate production in adipose tissue: a regulated function with extra-adipose implications. FASEB J 1992; 6(7):2405–2412.

51. Kim KH, Tae HJ. Pattern and regulation of acetyl-CoA carboxylase gene expression. J Nutr 1994; 124(8 suppl):1273S–1283S.

52. Assimacopoulos-Jeannet F, Brichard S, Rencurel F, et al. In vivo effects of hyperinsulinemia on lipogenic enzymes and glucose transporter expression in rat liver and adipose tissues. Metabolism 1995; 44(2):228–233.

53. Kehlenbrink S, Tonelli J, Koppaka S, et al. Inhibiting gluconeogenesis prevents fatty acid-induced increases in endogenous glucose production. Am J Physiol Endocrinol Metab 2009; 297(1):E165–E173.

54. Steppan CM, Bailey ST, Bhat S, et al. The hormone resistin links obesity to diabetes. Nature 2001; 409(6818):307–312.

55. Graveleau C, Zaha VG, Mohajer A, et al. Mouse and human resistins impair glucose transport in primary mouse cardiomyocytes, and oligomerization is required for this biological action. J Biol Chem 2005; 280(36):31679–31685.

56. Klein J, Permana PA, Owecki M, et al. What are subcutaneous adipocytes really good for? Exp Dermatol 2007; 16(1):45–70.

57. Zhang Y, Proenca R, Maffei M, et al. Positional cloning of the mouse obese gene and its human homologue. Nature 1994; 372(6505):425–432.

58. Hube F, Lietz U, Igel M, et al. Difference in leptin mRNA levels between omental and subcutaneous abdominal adipose tissue from obese humans. Horm Metab Res 1996; 28(12):690–693.

59. Friedman JM. The function of leptin in nutrition, weight, and physiology. Nutr Rev 2002; 60(10 pt 2):S1–S14.

60. Hoggard N, Mercer JG, Rayner DV, et al. Localization of leptin receptor mRNA splice variants in murine peripheral tissues by RT-PCR and in situ hybridization. Biochem Biophys Res Commun 1997; 232(2):383–387.

61. Ahima RS, Osei SY. Leptin signaling. Physiol Behav 2004; 81(2):223–241.

62. Toyoshima Y, Gavrilova O, Yakar S, et al. Leptin improves insulin resistance and hyperglycemia in a mouse model of type 2 diabetes. Endocrinology 2005; 146(9): 4024–4035.

63. Emilsson V, Liu YL, Cawthorne MA, et al. Expression of the functional leptin receptor mRNA in pancreatic islets and direct inhibitory action of leptin on insulin secretion. Diabetes 1997; 46(2):313–316.
64. Minokoshi Y, Kim YB, Peroni OD, et al. Leptin stimulates fatty-acid oxidation by activating AMP-activated protein kinase. Nature 2002; 415(6869):339–343.
65. Nogalska A, Sucajtys-Szulc E, Swierczynski J. Leptin decreases lipogenic enzyme gene expression through modification of SREBP-1c gene expression in white adipose tissue of aging rats. Metabolism 2005; 54(8):1041–1047.
66. Nakata M, Yada T, Soejima N, et al. Leptin promotes aggregation of human platelets via the long form of its receptor. Diabetes 1999; 48(2):426–429.
67. Bouloumie A, Drexler HC, Lafontan M, et al. Leptin, the product of Ob gene, promotes angiogenesis. Circ Res 1998; 83(10):1059–1066.
68. Fernandez-Riejos P, Goberna R, Sanchez-Margalet V. Leptin promotes cell survival and activates Jurkat T lymphocytes by stimulation of mitogen-activated protein kinase. Clin Exp Immunol 2008; 151(3):505–518.
69. Najib S, Sanchez-Margalet V. Human leptin promotes survival of human circulating blood monocytes prone to apoptosis by activation of p42/44 MAPK pathway. Cell Immunol 2002; 220(2):143–149.
70. Loffreda S, Yang SQ, Lin HZ, et al. Leptin regulates proinflammatory immune responses. FASEB J 1998; 12(1):57–65.
71. Sanchez-Margalet V, Martin-Romero C, Santos-Alvarez J, et al. Role of leptin as an immunomodulator of blood mononuclear cells: mechanisms of action. Clin Exp Immunol 2003; 133(1):11–19.
72. Murad A, Nath AK, Cha ST, et al. Leptin is an autocrine/paracrine regulator of wound healing. FASEB J 2003; 17(13):1895–1897.
73. Hotta K, Funahashi T, Arita Y, et al. Plasma concentrations of a novel, adipose-specific protein, adiponectin, in type 2 diabetic patients. Arterioscler Thromb Vasc Biol 2000; 20(6):1595–1599.
74. Arita Y, Kihara S, Ouchi N, et al. Paradoxical decrease of an adipose-specific protein, adiponectin, in obesity. Biochem Biophys Res Commun 1999; 257(1):79–83.
75. Yamauchi T, Kamon J, Ito Y, et al. Cloning of adiponectin receptors that mediate antidiabetic metabolic effects. Nature 2003; 423(6941):762–769.
76. Yamauchi T, Kamon J, Minokoshi Y, et al. Adiponectin stimulates glucose utilization and fatty-acid oxidation by activating AMP-activated protein kinase. Nat Med 2002; 8(11):1288–1295.
77. Ouchi N, Kihara S, Arita Y, et al. Novel modulator for endothelial adhesion molecules: adipocyte-derived plasma protein adiponectin. Circulation 1999; 100(25): 2473–2476.
78. Yokota T, Oritani K, Takahashi I, et al. Adiponectin, a new member of the family of soluble defense collagens, negatively regulates the growth of myelomonocytic progenitors and the functions of macrophages. Blood 2000; 96(5):1723–1732.
79. Tian L, Luo N, Klein RL, et al. Adiponectin reduces lipid accumulation in macrophage foam cells. Atherosclerosis 2009; 202(1):152–161.
80. Tsubakio-Yamamoto K, Matsuura F, Koseki M, et al. Adiponectin prevents atherosclerosis by increasing cholesterol efflux from macrophages. Biochem Biophys Res Commun 2008; 375(3):390–394.

81. Masaki T, Chiba S, Tatsukawa H, et al. Adiponectin protects LPS-induced liver injury through modulation of TNF-alpha in KK-Ay obese mice. Hepatology 2004; 40(1):177–184.
82. Kumada M, Kihara S, Ouchi N, et al. Adiponectin specifically increased tissue inhibitor of metalloproteinase-1 through interleukin-10 expression in human macrophages. Circulation 2004; 109(17):2046–2049.
83. Wolf AM, Wolf D, Rumpold H, et al. Adiponectin induces the anti-inflammatory cytokines IL-10 and IL-1RA in human leukocytes. Biochem Biophys Res Commun 2004; 323(2):630–635.
84. Rajala MW, Obici S, Scherer PE, et al. Adipose-derived resistin and gut-derived resistin-like molecule-beta selectively impair insulin action on glucose production. J Clin Invest 2003; 111(2):225–230.
85. Savage DB, Sewter CP, Klenk ES, et al. Resistin/Fizz3 expression in relation to obesity and peroxisome proliferator-activated receptor-gamma action in humans. Diabetes 2001; 50(10):2199–2202.
86. Janke J, Engeli S, Gorzelniak K, et al. Resistin gene expression in human adipocytes is not related to insulin resistance. Obes Res 2002; 10(1):1–5.
87. Burnett MS, Lee CW, Kinnaird TD, et al. The potential role of resistin in atherogenesis. Atherosclerosis 2005; 182(2):241–248.
88. Reilly MP, Lehrke M, Wolfe ML, et al. Resistin is an inflammatory marker of atherosclerosis in humans. Circulation 2005; 111(7):932–939.
89. Chu S, Ding W, Li K, et al. Plasma resistin associated with myocardium injury in patients with acute coronary syndrome. Circ J 2008; 72(8):1249–1253.
90. Verma S, Li SH, Wang CH, et al. Resistin promotes endothelial cell activation: further evidence of adipokine-endothelial interaction. Circulation 2003; 108(6): 736–740.
91. Kawanami D, Maemura K, Takeda N, et al. Direct reciprocal effects of resistin and adiponectin on vascular endothelial cells: a new insight into adipocytokine-endothelial cell interactions. Biochem Biophys Res Commun 2004; 314(2):415–419.
92. Senolt L, Housa D, Vernerova Z, et al. Resistin in rheumatoid arthritis synovial tissue, synovial fluid and serum. Ann Rheum Dis 2007; 66(4):458–463.
93. Gonzalez-Gay MA, Garcia-Unzueta MT, Gonzalez-Juanatey C, et al. Anti-TNF-alpha therapy modulates resistin in patients with rheumatoid arthritis. Clin Exp Rheumatol 2008; 26(2):311–316.
94. Almehed K, d'Elia HF, Bokarewa M, et al. Role of resistin as a marker of inflammation in systemic lupus erythematosus. Arthritis Res Ther 2008; 10(1):R15.
95. Johnston A, Arnadottir S, Gudjonsson JE, et al. Obesity in psoriasis: leptin and resistin as mediators of cutaneous inflammation. Br J Dermatol 2008; 159(2):342–350.
96. Konrad A, Lehrke M, Schachinger V, et al. Resistin is an inflammatory marker of inflammatory bowel disease in humans. Eur J Gastroenterol Hepatol 2007; 19(12): 1070–1074.
97. Weisberg SP, McCann D, Desai M, et al. Obesity is associated with macrophage accumulation in adipose tissue. J Clin Invest 2003; 112(12):1796–1808.
98. Hotamisligil GS, Shargill NS, Spiegelman BM. Adipose expression of tumor necrosis factor-alpha: direct role in obesity-linked insulin resistance. Science 1993; 259(5091):87–91.

99. Hotamisligil GS, Arner P, Caro JF, et al. Increased adipose tissue expression of tumor necrosis factor-alpha in human obesity and insulin resistance. J Clin Invest 1995; 95(5):2409–2415.

100. Hotamisligil GS. The role of TNFalpha and TNF receptors in obesity and insulin resistance. J Intern Med 1999; 245(6):621–625.

101. Green A, Dobias SB, Walters DJ, et al. Tumor necrosis factor increases the rate of lipolysis in primary cultures of adipocytes without altering levels of hormone-sensitive lipase. Endocrinology 1994; 134(6):2581–2588.

102. Ruan H, Hacohen N, Golub TR, et al. Tumor necrosis factor-alpha suppresses adipocyte-specific genes and activates expression of preadipocyte genes in 3T3-L1 adipocytes: nuclear factor-kappaB activation by TNF-alpha is obligatory. Diabetes 2002; 51(5):1319–1336.

103. Feingold KR, Grunfeld C. Role of cytokines in inducing hyperlipidemia. Diabetes 1992; 41(suppl 2):97–101.

104. Peraldi P, Hotamisligil GS, Buurman WA, et al. Tumor necrosis factor (TNF)-alpha inhibits insulin signaling through stimulation of the p55 TNF receptor and activation of sphingomyelinase. J Biol Chem 1996; 271(22):13018–13022.

105. Wang B, Jenkins JR, Trayhurn P. Expression and secretion of inflammation-related adipokines by human adipocytes differentiated in culture: integrated response to TNF-alpha. Am J Physiol Endocrinol Metab 2005; 288(4):E731–E740.

106. Ofei F, Hurel S, Newkirk J, et al. Effects of an engineered human anti-TNF-alpha antibody (CDP571) on insulin sensitivity and glycemic control in patients with NIDDM. Diabetes 1996; 45(7):881–885.

107. Samad F, Yamamoto K, Pandey M, et al. Elevated expression of transforming growth factor-beta in adipose tissue from obese mice. Mol Med 1997; 3(1):37–48.

108. Samad F, Uysal KT, Wiesbrock SM, et al. Tumor necrosis factor alpha is a key component in the obesity-linked elevation of plasminogen activator inhibitor 1. Proc Natl Acad Sci U S A 1999; 96(12):6902–6907.

109. Oberkofler H, Dallinger G, Liu YM, et al. Uncoupling protein gene: quantification of expression levels in adipose tissues of obese and non-obese humans. J Lipid Res 1997; 38(10):2125–2133.

110. Lin CS, Klingenberg M. Isolation of the uncoupling protein from brown adipose tissue mitochondria. FEBS Lett 1980; 113(2):299–303.

111. Lowell BB, Spiegelman BM. Towards a molecular understanding of adaptive thermogenesis. Nature 2000; 404(6778):652–660.

112. Huttunen P, Hirvonen J, Kinnula V. The occurrence of brown adipose tissue in outdoor workers. Eur J Appl Physiol Occup Physiol 1981; 46(4):339–345.

113. Nedergaard J, Golozoubova V, Matthias A, et al. UCP1: the only protein able to mediate adaptive non-shivering thermogenesis and metabolic inefficiency. Biochim Biophys Acta 2001; 1504(1):82–106.

114. Klingenspor M. Cold-induced recruitment of brown adipose tissue thermogenesis. Exp Physiol 2003; 88(1):141–148.

115. Collins S, Cao W, Robidoux J. Learning new tricks from old dogs: beta-adrenergic receptors teach new lessons on firing up adipose tissue metabolism. Mol Endocrinol 2004; 18(9):2123–2131.

116. Lowell BB, S-Susulic V, Hamann A, et al. Development of obesity in transgenic mice after genetic ablation of brown adipose tissue. Nature 1993; 366(6457):740–742.

117. Klaus S, Munzberg H, Truloff C, et al. Physiology of transgenic mice with brown fat ablation: obesity is due to lowered body temperature. Am J Physiol 1998; 274(2 pt 2):R287–R293.

118. Oppert JM, Vohl MC, Chagnon M, et al. DNA polymorphism in the uncoupling protein (UCP) gene and human body fat. Int J Obes Relat Metab Disord 1994; 18(8): 526–531.

119. Walston J, Silver K, Bogardus C, et al. Time of onset of non-insulin-dependent diabetes mellitus and genetic variation in the beta 3-adrenergic-receptor gene. N Engl J Med 1995; 333(6):343–347.

120. Evans D, Minouchehr S, Hagemann G, et al. Frequency of and interaction between polymorphisms in the beta3-adrenergic receptor and in uncoupling proteins 1 and 2 and obesity in Germans. Int J Obes Relat Metab Disord 2000; 24(10):1239–1245.

121. Warden C. Genetics of uncoupling proteins in humans. Int J Obes Relat Metab Disord 1999; 23(suppl 6):S46–S48.

122. Himms-Hagen J. Exercise in a pill: feasibility of energy expenditure targets. Curr Drug Targets CNS Neurol Disord 2004; 3(5):389–409.

123. Ogden CL, Carroll MD, Curtin LR, et al. Prevalence of overweight and obesity in the United States, 1999–2004. JAMA 2006; 295(13):1549–1555.

124. Yusuf S, Hawken S, Ounpuu S, et al. Obesity and the risk of myocardial infarction in 27,000 participants from 52 countries: a case-control study. Lancet 2005; 366 (9497):1640–1649.

125. Alberti KG, Eckel RH, Grundy SM, et al. Harmonizing the metabolic syndrome: a joint interim statement of the International Diabetes Federation Task Force on Epidemiology and Prevention; National Heart, Lung, and Blood Institute; American Heart Association; World Heart Federation; International Atherosclerosis Society; and International Association for the Study of Obesity. Circulation 2009; 120(16):1640–1645.

126. Permana PA, Menge C, Reaven PD. Macrophage-secreted factors induce adipocyte inflammation and insulin resistance. Biochem Biophys Res Commun 2006; 341(2): 507–514.

127. Suganami T, Tanimoto-Koyama K, Nishida J, et al. Role of the Toll-like receptor 4/NF-kappaB pathway in saturated fatty acid-induced inflammatory changes in the interaction between adipocytes and macrophages. Arterioscler Thromb Vasc Biol 2007; 27(1):84–91.

128. Myers MG, Cowley MA, Munzberg H. Mechanisms of leptin action and leptin resistance. Annu Rev Physiol 2008; 70:537–556.

129. Niswender KD, Baskin DG, Schwartz MW. Insulin and its evolving partnership with leptin in the hypothalamic control of energy homeostasis. Trends Endocrinol Metab 2004; 15(8):362–369.

130. Hegele RA, Joy TR, Al-Attar SA, et al. Lipodystrophies: windows on adipose biology and metabolism. J Lipid Res 2007; 48(7):1433–1444.

131. Garg A, Agarwal AK. Lipodystrophies: disorders of adipose tissue biology. Biochim Biophys Acta 2009; 1791(6):507–513.

132. Carr A, Samaras K, Burton S, et al. A syndrome of peripheral lipodystrophy, hyperlipidaemia and insulin resistance in patients receiving HIV protease inhibitors. AIDS 1998; 12(7):F51–F58.

133. Carr A. HIV lipodystrophy: risk factors, pathogenesis, diagnosis and management. AIDS 2003; 17(suppl 1):S141–S148.

134. Grinspoon S, Carr A. Cardiovascular risk and body-fat abnormalities in HIV-infected adults. N Engl J Med 2005; 352(1):48–62.

135. James J, Carruthers A, Carruthers J. HIV-associated facial lipoatrophy. Dermatol Surg 2002; 28(11):979–986.

136. Leow MK, Addy CL, Mantzoros CS. Human immunodeficiency virus/highly active antiretroviral therapy-associated metabolic syndrome: clinical presentation, pathophysiology, and therapeutic strategies. J Clin Endocrinol Metab 2003; 88(5):1961–1976.

137. Jan V, Cervera P, Maachi M, et al. Altered fat differentiation and adipocytokine expression are inter-related and linked to morphological changes and insulin resistance in HIV-1-infected lipodystrophic patients. Antivir Ther 2004; 9(4):555–564.

138. Domingo P, Matias-Guiu X, Pujol RM, et al. Subcutaneous adipocyte apoptosis in HIV-1 protease inhibitor-associated lipodystrophy. AIDS 1999; 13(16):2261–2267.

139. Carr A, Samaras K, Chisholm DJ, et al. Pathogenesis of HIV-1-protease inhibitor-associated peripheral lipodystrophy, hyperlipidaemia, and insulin resistance. Lancet 1998; 351(9119):1881–1883.

140. Caron M, Auclair M, Sterlingot H, et al. Some HIV protease inhibitors alter lamin A/C maturation and stability, SREBP-1 nuclear localization and adipocyte differentiation. AIDS 2003; 17(17):2437–2444.

141. Caron M, Auclair M, Lagathu C, et al. The HIV-1 nucleoside reverse transcriptase inhibitors stavudine and zidovudine alter adipocyte functions in vitro. AIDS 2004; 18(16):2127–2136.

142. Lewis W, Kohler JJ, Hosseini SH, et al. Antiretroviral nucleosides, deoxynucleotide carrier and mitochondrial DNA: evidence supporting the DNA pol gamma hypothesis. AIDS 2006; 20(5):675–684.

143. Lagathu C, Bastard JP, Auclair M, et al. Antiretroviral drugs with adverse effects on adipocyte lipid metabolism and survival alter the expression and secretion of proinflammatory cytokines and adiponectin in vitro. Antivir Ther 2004; 9(6):911–920.

144. Jones SP, Janneh O, Back DJ, et al. Altered adipokine response in murine 3T3-F442A adipocytes treated with protease inhibitors and nucleoside reverse transcriptase inhibitors. Antivir Ther 2005; 10(2):207–213.

145. Lagathu C, Eustace B, Prot M, et al. Some HIV antiretrovirals increase oxidative stress and alter chemokine, cytokine or adiponectin production in human adipocytes and macrophages. Antivir Ther 2007; 12(4):489–500.

146. Bertrand HA, Masoro EJ, Yu BP. Increasing adipocyte number as the basis for perirenal depot growth in adult rats. Science 1978; 201(4362):1234–1235.

147. Kirkland JL, Tchkonia T, Pirtskhalava T, et al. Adipogenesis and aging: does aging make fat go MAD? Exp Gerontol 2002; 37(6):757–767.

148. Coleman S, Saboeiro A, Sengelmann R. A comparison of lipoatrophy and aging: volume deficits in the face. Aesthetic Plast Surg 2009; 33(1):14–21.

149. Kuk JL, Saunders TJ, Davidson LE, et al. Age-related changes in total and regional fat distribution. Ageing Res Rev 2009; 8(4):339–348.

150. Stevens J, Cai J, Pamuk ER, et al. The effect of age on the association between body-mass index and mortality. N Engl J Med 1998; 338(1):1–7.

151. Visscher TL, Seidell JC, Molarius A, et al. A comparison of body mass index, waist-hip ratio and waist circumference as predictors of all-cause mortality among

the elderly: the Rotterdam study. Int J Obes Relat Metab Disord 2001; 25(11): 1730–1735.

152. Djian P, Roncari AK, Hollenberg CH. Influence of anatomic site and age on the replication and differentiation of rat adipocyte precursors in culture. J Clin Invest 1983; 72(4):1200–1208.

153. Kirkland JL, Hollenberg CH, Gillon WS. Age, anatomic site, and the replication and differentiation of adipocyte precursors. Am J Physiol 1990; 258(2 pt 1):C206–C210.

154. Kirkland JL, Hollenberg CH, Kindler S, et al. Effects of age and anatomic site on preadipocyte number in rat fat depots. J Gerontol 1994; 49(1):B31–B35.

155. Kirkland JL, Dobson DE. Preadipocyte function and aging: links between age-related changes in cell dynamics and altered fat tissue function. J Am Geriatr Soc 1997; 45(8):959–967.

156. Karagiannides I, Tchkonia T, Dobson DE, et al. Altered expression of C/EBP family members results in decreased adipogenesis with aging. Am J Physiol Regul Integr Comp Physiol 2001; 280(6):R1772–R1780.

157. Miard S, Dombrowski L, Carter S, et al. Aging alters PPARgamma in rodent and human adipose tissue by modulating the balance in steroid receptor coactivator-1. Aging Cell 2009; 8(4):449–459.

158. Karagiannides I, Thomou T, Tchkonia T, et al. Increased CUG triplet repeat-binding protein-1 predisposes to impaired adipogenesis with aging. J Biol Chem 2006; 281(32):23025–23033.

159. Tchkonia T, Pirtskhalava T, Thomou T, et al. Increased TNFalpha and CCAAT/enhancer-binding protein homologous protein with aging predispose preadipocytes to resist adipogenesis. Am J Physiol Endocrinol Metab 2007; 293(6):E1810–E1819.

160. Cartwright MJ, Tchkonia T, Kirkland JL. Aging in adipocytes: potential impact of inherent, depot-specific mechanisms. Exp Gerontol 2007; 42(6):463–471.

161. El-Jack AK, Hamm JK, Pilch PF, et al. Reconstitution of insulin-sensitive glucose transport in fibroblasts requires expression of both PPARgamma and C/EBPalpha. J Biol Chem 1999; 274(12):7946–7951.

162. Caserta F, Tchkonia T, Civelek VN, et al. Fat depot origin affects fatty acid handling in cultured rat and human preadipocytes. Am J Physiol Endocrinol Metab 2001; 280(2):E238–E247.

163. Morin CL, Gayles EC, Podolin DA, et al. Adipose tissue-derived tumor necrosis factor activity correlates with fat cell size but not insulin action in aging rats. Endocrinology 1998; 139(12):4998–5005.

164. Rohrich RJ, Pessa JE. The fat compartments of the face: anatomy and clinical implications for cosmetic surgery. Plast Reconstr Surg 2007; 119(7):2219–2227.

3

Benign and malignant neoplasms

Pritesh S. Karia, Wael A. Ghattas, Javad Beheshti, Clay J. Cockerell,
and Chrysalyne D. Schmults

INTRODUCTION

Adipose tissue tumors are the most common soft tissue tumors. They can occur at any age and in almost any anatomic location. The vast majority of adipocytic tumors are benign lipomas and are easily diagnosed and treated. However, beyond lipomas, identification of other types of benign and malignant adipocytic tumors can be challenging. Misdiagnosis can lead to ineffective treatment and related comorbidities. Therefore, it is critical to fully understand the clinical manifestations of adipocytic tumors in order to provide optimal patient care. This chapter summarizes clinical features, prognosis, and treatment of some of the most common benign and malignant adipocytic tumors.

BACKGROUND

Adipose tissue is connective tissue consisting mainly of fat cells, or adipocytes, which store cellular energy in the form of triglycerides. It is primarily found as a continuous layer under the skin, beneath abdominal muscles, and surrounding organs such as the heart and kidneys. As described in the previous chapter, in addition to serving as the main reservoir of energy, adipose tissue plays an important role in providing mechanical and thermal support, as well as in insulin regulation, secretion of endocrine hormones, and in physiological processes such as inflammation.

The two major types of adipose tissue are white adipose tissue (WAT) and brown adipose tissue (BAT). The predominant form of adipose tissue found in humans is WAT and it is concentrated in the abdomen and beneath the skin (1). BAT is primarily found in infants and serves the important function of generating heat through nonshivering thermogenesis. In adults, BAT is minimal and is found mainly in small tissue islands within the thorax.

Considerable research is currently being conducted in the field of adipocyte cell cycle and adipogenesis, as described in chapter 1. These ongoing investigations will likely shed additional light on the pathogenesis of benign and malignant tumors described herein.

CURRENT STATE OF KNOWLEDGE

Benign Neoplasms of Adipose Tissue

A vast majority of soft tissue tumors, including adipocytic tumors, are benign with very high cure rates after surgical excision. At present, the 2002 World Health Organization (WHO) Classification of Soft Tissue Tumors divides benign tumors of adipose tissue into the following categories: lipoma, lipoma variants (including angiolipoma, chondroid lipoma, and spindle cell/pleomorphic lipoma), lipoblastoma/lipoblastomatosis, myolipoma, extra-adrenal myelolipoma, extrarenal angiomyolipoma, lipomatosis of nerve, lipomatosis, and hibernoma (2).

These tumors can be more easily divided into five distinct groups to provide a conceptually convenient categorization for diagnosis and management. These categories are summarized in Table 3.1 and include the following:

1. Lipoma and its histological variants: tumors composed of mature fat, which can be further classified as superficial or deep and single or multiple. Histological variants include angiolipoma, chondroid lipoma, and spindle cell/pleiomorphic lipoma. Patients with multiple lesions may have benign familial lipomatosis.
2. Other adipose tumors: tumors that differ from lipomas with regard to their clinical presentation, deeper anatomic location, and microscopic appearance. They include lipoblastoma/lipoblastomatosis, myolipoma, extra-adrenal myelolipoma, and extrarenal angiomyolipoma.
3. Lipomatous tumors: tumors composed of adipocytes but arising within nonadipose tissues, such as lipomatosis of nerve.
4. Infiltrating lipomas: diffuse proliferative adipose tumors that compress surrounding structures, such as the lipomatosis disorders (3).
5. Hibernoma: a tumor composed of BAT.

LIPOMA AND ITS HISTOLOGICAL VARIANTS

Lipoma and its histological variants are benign lesions that usually occur in adults. They are composed of a mature adipose tissue and often manifest as painless mobile doughy soft tissue masses, palpable below the skin (Figs. 3.1 and 3.2). They are characterized by their anatomic location as either

Table 3.1 Benign Neoplasms of Adipose Tissue

Tumor type	Clinical features	Prognosis and treatment
Lipoma and its histological variants		
Lipoma	– Painless mass with characteristic doughy feel – Subcutaneous (most commonly) or deep – Subcutaneous lesions <5 cm – Deep lesions often >5 cm – More common in obese people – Uncommon in children	– Surgical excision or liposuction – 1%–4% may recur
Angiolipoma	– Similar to lipoma but with a vascular proliferative component in addition to the adipocyte proliferation – Common in young males 20–30 years old – Often tender	– Surgical excision, rare local recurrence
Chondroid lipoma	– Rare tumor in subcutaneous or deeper soft tissues – Tumor has a myxochondroid stromal background – Predominantly found in women	– Surgical excision, rare local recurrence
Spindle cell/pleomorphic lipoma	– Tumor composed of both adipocytes and spindle cells – More common in men	– Surgical excision, rare local recurrence
Benign familial lipomatosis	– Multiple lipomas (20–100) in individuals with family history of similar tumors – Autosomal dominant because of mutations of chromosome 12q15 that encodes the high-mobility group protein isoform 1-C (HMGIC)	– Surgical excision can be used, although often impractical because of numerous tumors – Liposuction or other fat-ablative techniques may be more feasible

(Continued)

Table 3.1 Benign Neoplasms of Adipose Tissue (*Continued*)

Tumor type	Clinical features	Prognosis and treatment
Other adipose tumors *Lipoblastoma/ Lipoblastomatosis*	– Fetal adipose tissue tumors – Common in children <3 years – More common in males – Circumscribed lesions = lipoblastoma – Diffuse lesions = lipoblastomatosis – Distribution: extremities (common), neck, abdomen, mediastinum, retroperitoneum	– Local excision without radical resection – 14%–25% may recur
Myolipoma	– Rare. Because of proliferation of fat and smooth muscle tissue – Found in adults 50–60 years old – More common in women – Distribution: retroperitoneum, abdomen	– Surgical excision with low recurrence
Extra-adrenal myelolipoma	– Very rare tumor composed of fat cells and bone marrow cells – Common in retroperitoneum and pelvic region – More common in women >40 years	– Surgical excision
Extrarenal angiomyolipoma	– Very rare tumor composed of fat cells, smooth muscle, and blood vessels – Most commonly found in liver	– Surgical excision

Lipomatous tumors

Lipomatosis of Nerve	– Gradually enlarging mass with neurological symptoms – Patients often present before the age of 30 – Median and ulnar nerves most commonly affected – Upper extremity affected in majority of cases	– No effective treatment – Amputation for patients with macrodactyly
Infiltrating lipomas/Lipomatosis	– Notable accumulation of fat in affected areas – Diffuse lipomatosis common in children <2 years. Distribution: trunk, extremities, head and neck, pelvis – Pelvic lipomatosis common in black males – Multiple lipomatosis common in middle-aged men with history of liver disease or high alcohol consumption, mainly on the neck – Steroid lipomatosis common in hormone therapy patients (Addisonian facies, buffalo hump)	– Palliative surgical removal – Often recurs after surgery
Hibernoma	– Rare tumor involving brown adipose tissue – Mobile mass, feels warm on physical examination – Mainly in adults 30–40 years old – Distribution: deep thorax, upper back	– Surgical excision usually curative

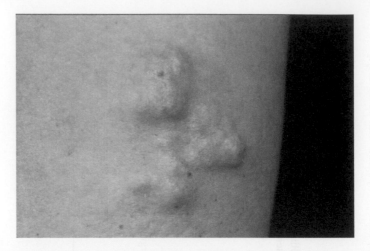

Figure 3.1 Lipomas usually present with soft mobile subcutaneous lumps.

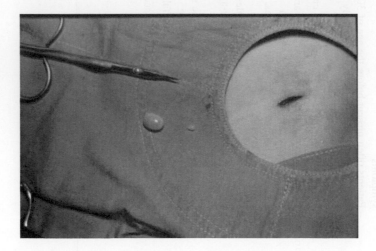

Figure 3.2 Mobile encapsulated lipoma. A variant with a thin capsule that may be shelled out in contrast to other lipomas which are more diffuse.

subcutaneous or deep and are not distinguishable histologically from normal fat; however, grossly they appear pale yellow to orange with a greasy surface (Figs. 3.3–3.5) (3). Subcutaneous lipomas are far more common as compared to deep lipomas, which account for about 1% of all cases. However, deep lipomas

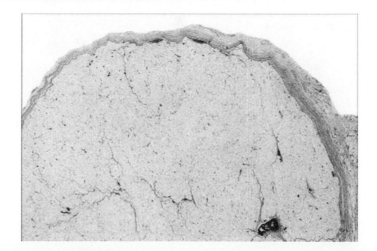

Figure 3.3 Subcutaneous lipoma composed of mature lobules of adipose tissue. The thin capsule is discernible at the deep tissue surface. (H&E), original magnification 40x.

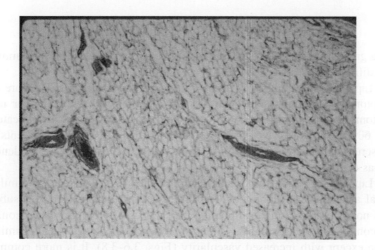

Figure 3.4 Mature adipose tissue in a lipoma. Feeding vessels are scattered throughout. (H&E), original magnification 100x.

may not be clinically apparent and may thus go undiagnosed. Lesions are often located on the trunk and extremities and are unusual in the hand and foot (3,4). Most lipomas are less than 5 cm in diameter and can easily be removed by surgical excision or liposuction with a very low risk of recurrence. Deep lipomas

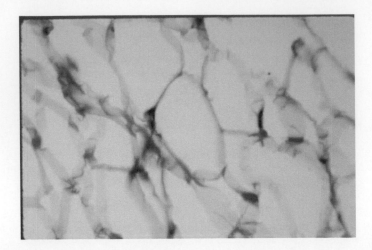

Figure 3.5 Mature adipocytes (fat cells) in lipoma. The cells have few large vacuoles (or more commonly one vacuole) of fat in their cytoplasm that push the nuclei to the periphery. In the center, two darkly stained crescent-shaped nuclei are seen that are pushed to the periphery against the cell membranes. (H&E), original magnification 400x.

have a greater tendency to recur, probably because complete surgical removal is more difficult (5).

Lipomas most commonly occur in men in their 40s to 60s. They are often asymptomatic, although some patients may report local tenderness or neural symptoms because of compression of peripheral nerves (4). Studies indicate that about 60% of lipomas have chromosomal abnormalities. As well, patients with high serum cholesterol levels and diabetic patients have a higher incidence of lipomas (5).

Lipoma has three important histological variants, which are similar in clinical appearance to lipoma and present as asymptomatic or tender subcutaneous nodules. Like ordinary lipomas, they are usually cured by excision. The most common of these variants is angiolipoma, which is histologically similar to lipoma except with increased vascularity (Figs. 3.6–3.8). It is more commonly tender than ordinary lipomas. Angiolipoma is most common in young men in their teens and 20s, with more than 70% being located on the trunk and extremities (6).

Chondroid lipoma is a rare histological variant of lipoma. It is most common in women and is located in the proximal extremities (particularly groin and shoulder regions). Histologically, the tumors consist of strands and nests of adipocytes, but, in contrast to lipoma, within a myxochondroid or hyalinized background (5).

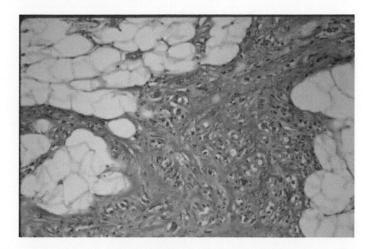

Figure 3.6 Angiolipoma showing an admixture of mature adipose tissue and numerous well-formed small vessels. (H&E), original magnification 200x.

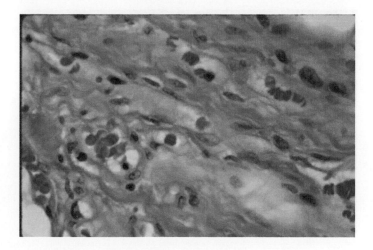

Figure 3.7 Angiolipoma: higher power view shows the well-formed vessels containing red blood cells. (H&E), original magnification 400x.

Spindle cell or pleomorphic lipoma is most common in men aged 30 to 60, mainly on posterior neck and shoulder (Fig. 3.9) (2,6). Microscopically, these lesions are usually composed of a relatively equal ratio of fat and spindle cells (Figs. 3.10–3.12) (6).

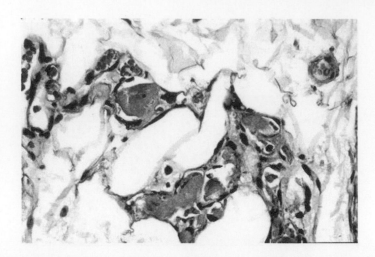

Figure 3.8 Thrombosis frequently seen within vessels in angiolipoma. (H&E), original magnification 400x.

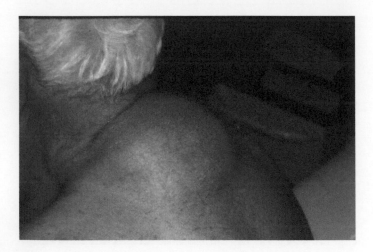

Figure 3.9 Spindle cell lipoma. Usually seen in mid to late adulthood in males, 80% of tumors occur in back of the neck, upper back, and shoulder areas.

Benign familial lipomatosis is the occurrence of multiple lipomas (ordinary lipoma and its subtypes) in individuals with a family history of similar tumors. It is autosomal dominant and results from alterations in chromosome 12q15, which encodes the high-mobility group protein isoform I-C (HMGIC).

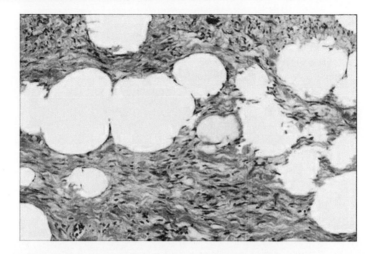

Figure 3.10 Spindle cell lipoma: an admixture of mature adipose tissue, bland spindle cells, and thick collagen bundles. (H&E), original magnification 200x.

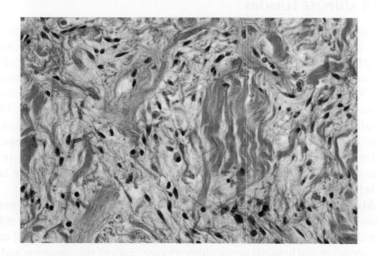

Figure 3.11 Spindle cell lipoma: an admixture of bland spindle cells and thick collagen bundles. Infiltrating mast cells and myxoid background are frequently seen as visible in this tumor. (H&E), original magnification 400x.

Bothersome tumors can be surgically excised. However, since patients may have 20 to 100 tumors, excision of all lesions is usually too cumbersome to attempt surgically. Liposuction and new technologies involving deeply penetrating light sources, described in subsequent, may be considered for these patients.

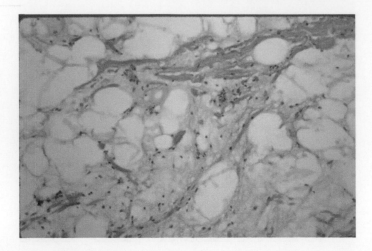

Figure 3.12 Myxoid change more pronounced in this spindle cell lipoma. (H&E), original magnification 200x.

OTHER ADIPOSE TUMORS

Lipoblastoma/lipoblastomatosis is a rare tumor of fetal adipose tissue that occurs in infancy and early childhood. Lipoblastoma is used to describe circumscribed lesions, whereas lipoblastomatosis is used to describe diffuse infiltrating lesions (6). These tumors are three to four times more common in males. They are often located in the superficial soft tissues of the extremities, and also occur in the abdomen, mediastinum, and retroperitoneum (7). Microscopically, the tumors are composed of fat lobules separated by fibrous connective tissue (Fig. 3.13). Lipoblastoma/lipoblastomatosis can be treated by complete local excision. However, recurrence is very common in lipoblastomatosis, since tumor margins are often less well defined in these larger, more infiltrative tumors (3).

Myolipoma is an extremely rare tumor caused by proliferation of both fat and smooth muscle tissue. It occurs in adults, usually aged 40 to 50, and is twice as common in women as in men. It is typically located in the abdominal cavity, retroperitoneum and inguinal areas, although rare cases of subcutaneous and deep soft tissue tumors have been reported on the trunk and extremities (Fig. 3.14) (6). Tumors are often large, measuring 10 to 25 cm in diameter. Histologically, these tumors have a variable mixture of smooth muscle and adipose tissue, although the smooth muscle component typically predominates (6). Lesions can be removed by surgical excision, usually with no local recurrence.

Extra-adrenal myelolipoma and extrarenal angiomyolipoma are extremely rare adipose tumors. Extra-adrenal myelolipoma is composed of mature adipose

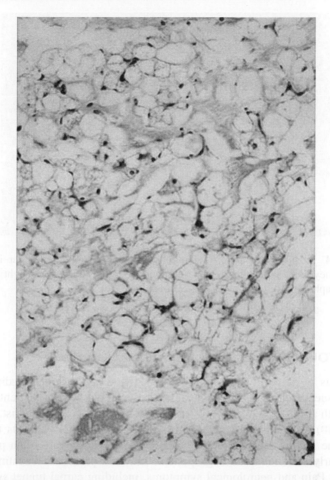

Figure 3.13 Lipoblastoma: an admixture of mature adipocytes and multivacuolated lipoblasts. Myxoid stroma and plexiform vasculature are also seen. (H&E), original magnification 200x.

tissue with some hematopoietic component. It is predominantly found in adults over the age of 40 years and is more common in females. Lesions are often solitary 4- to 15-cm masses in the retroperitoneum or within the pelvis (8). Extrarenal angiomyolipoma is composed of mature fat cells, smooth muscle cells, and thick-walled blood vessels (Fig. 3.15). These tumors are common in middle-aged women, mainly affecting the liver and other organs such as the skin (9). The treatment for both extra-adrenal myelolipoma and extrarenal angiomyolipoma is surgical excision.

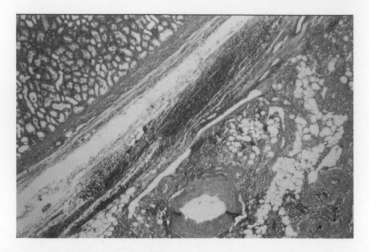

Figure 3.14 Angiomyolipomas. Angiomyolipomas most commonly occur in kidney. Normal kidney tissue is seen in the upper left and the tumor in the lower right portion of the photograph. (H&E), original magnification 100x.

LIPOMATOUS TUMORS (LIPOMATOSIS OF NERVE)

Lipomatosis of nerve involves the invasion of the epineurium by adipose and fibrous tissue, resulting in nerve entanglement and enlargement. Patients usually present with a soft, slowly growing mass of the volar aspect of the wrist, hand, or forearm (10). Median nerve involvement is most common, whereas the ulnar nerve is the second most commonly affected site. Tumors are often present at birth or early childhood, although patients may not present for treatment until adulthood. Pain and neurological symptoms, including carpal tunnel syndrome, have been associated with lipomatosis of the nerve (6). On gross examination of the resected tumor, the affected nerves are enlarged by infiltrations of yellow fibrofatty tissues. When viewed under the microscope, nerve bundles are separated by this infiltrating tissue. The nerve fibers themselves may appear normal. However, neuronal atrophy may be observed in late stages of the disease. Macrodactyly is observed in most cases and is particularly common in females (6). No effective treatment is available for lipomatosis of the nerve. Resection generally results in severe nerve deficits and poor function. Amputation is often necessary.

INFILTRATING LIPOMAS/LIPOMATOSIS

Lipomatosis is a diffuse overgrowth of mature adipose tissue that can affect different anatomic regions of the body. There are several different types of

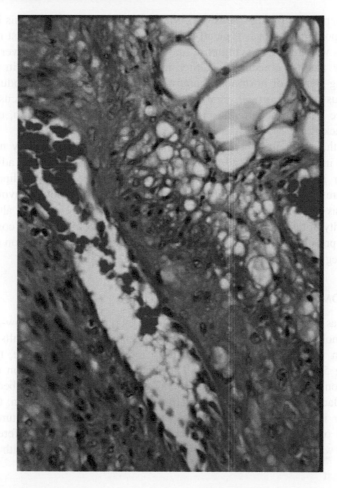

Figure 3.15 Angiomyolipoma: an admixture of mature adipose tissue, benign smooth muscle, and vessels. (H&E), original magnification 400x.

lipomatosis, such as diffuse lipomatosis, pelvic lipomatosis, symmetric lipomatosis, and steroid lipomatosis. Diffuse lipomatosis is common in children below the age of 2 years and typically involves the trunk or extremities. Patients have massive accumulation of fat in the affected areas (10). Pelvic lipomatosis is characterized by an overgrowth of fat in the perirectal and perivisceral areas, often leading to compression of the lower urinary tract. It is most commonly found in black males. Patients with pelvic lipomatosis may present with mild perineal pain and increased urinary frequency in early stages of the disease and hematuria, abdominal pain, constipation, nausea, and back pain in later stages of the disease (5). Multiple symmetric lipomatosis is a rare form of lipomatosis that is typically seen in middle-aged men. A vast majority of patients with multiple symmetric lipomatosis have a history of liver disease and heavy alcohol consumption. Steroid lipomatosis is common in patients undergoing steroid or hormonal therapy, or who have increased production of endogenous adrenocortical steroids. It is characterized by a cushingoid appearance with an accumulation of fat on the face, sternal region, or upper middle back (2).

All the different subtypes of lipomatosis can be diagnosed by magnetic resonance imaging (MRI) and confirmed by biopsy. Histologically, adipocytes are similar in appearance to normal fat cells. Differences between lipomatosis subtypes are only observed with regard to the site and distribution of involvement. Lipomatosis can be treated by palliative surgical removal of excess fat, although a vast majority of tumors recur after surgery, likely because of inability to completely resect the proliferating adipocytes. In some cases, massive accumulation of fat in the neck region can result in laryngeal obstruction and death (2).

HIBERNOMA

Hibernomas are rare tumors involving BAT. They often present as slow-growing painless mobile soft tissue masses on the upper back of young adults. Hibernomas can vary in color from tan to deep red and are fairly large, typically measuring 5 to 10 cm in diameter. They feel warm to the touch on physical examination because of BAT's ability to generate heat, as described in the section "Background." Although sometimes subcutaneous in location, they can also occur in the chest, where BAT persists into adulthood. The tumors are composed of lobules of adipose cells with varying degrees of differentiation consistent with BAT (Fig. 3.16) (6). Hibernomas are usually cured with surgical excision.

Malignant Neoplasms of Adipose Tissue

Malignant soft tissue tumors account for less than 1% of human malignancies. However, they are life-threatening and pose significant diagnostic and therapeutic challenges. Liposarcomas are a subset of malignant soft tissue sarcomas that arise from adipocytes. They comprise approximately 17% of soft tissue sarcomas and usually occur in adults in the extremities or abdominal/retroperitoneal regions (2). Since they can present to dermatologists as asymptomatic, enlarging, subcutaneous masses of the extremities or other locations, it is important to be familiar with their clinical manifestations, subtypes, and staging.

The 2002 WHO Classification of Soft Tissue Tumors divides malignant tumors of adipose tissue (liposarcomas) into the following six categories,

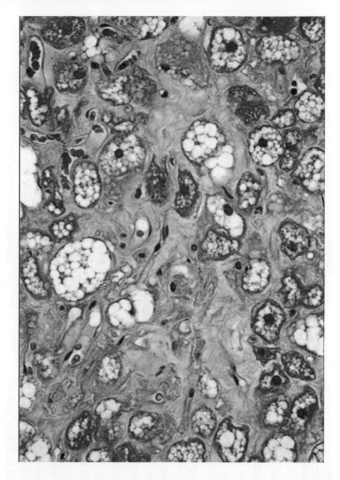

Figure 3.16 Hibernoma: sheets of large cells with central nuclei and eosinophilic granular cytoplasm. Some of the cells contain mature fat vacuoles. (H&E), original magnification 400x.

summarized in Table 3.2: myxoid, round cell, dedifferentiated, pleomorphic, mixed-type, and liposarcoma not otherwise specified (Figs. 3.17 and 3.18) (2).

Myxoid liposarcoma and round cell liposarcoma share a wide variety of clinical and morphological similarities. Myxoid liposarcoma is the most common subtype of liposarcoma accounting for about half of all cases. It is composed of a variable mixture of myxoid stroma, capillary networks, and proliferating lipoblasts (precursors of adipocytes that consist of lipid-filled vacuoles) with varying degrees of maturation (Figs. 3.19 and 3.20) (11). On the other hand, round cell liposarcoma is a very rare tumor that represents a poorly differentiated form of myxoid liposarcoma composed of rounded cells (likely

Table 3.2 Variants of Malignant Liposarcoma

Tumor type	Clinical features	Prognosis and treatment
Myxoid liposarcoma	– Most common subtype of liposarcoma – Lipoblasts in a myxoid stroma – Distribution: deep soft tissues of extremities	– Surgical excision, sometimes combined with radiation – Rarely metastasizes
Round cell liposarcoma	– A poorly differentiated form of myxoid liposarcoma – Distribution: deep soft tissues of extremities especially thighs and popliteal areas	– Surgical excision, sometimes combined with radiation – High chance of metastasis
Dedifferentiated liposarcoma	– Tumor composed of two distinct cell types: well-differentiated liposarcoma and nonlipogenic sarcoma – Distribution: most commonly in extremities, rare in neck and head	– Surgical excision, usually with adjuvant radiation and/or chemotherapy – 41% may recur – 17% may metastasize
Pleomorphic liposarcoma	– Rare tumor composed of pleomorphic lipoblasts – Distribution: limbs of older adults, but may also be found on trunk and retroperitoneum	– Surgical excision, usually with adjuvant radiation and/or chemotherapy – 28% recur, 44% metastasize – 50% mortality rate
Mixed-type liposarcoma	– Extremely rare form of liposarcoma comproed of various combinations of the above histological types – Often found in elderly patients – Distribution: intra-abdominal, retroperitoneum	– Surgical excision, usually with adjuvant radiation and/or chemotherapy – Prognosis depends upon tumor extent and histological composition

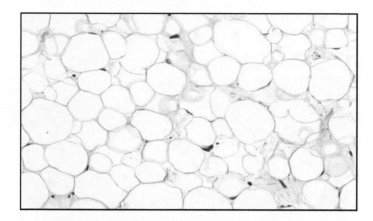

Figure 3.17 Well-differentiated liposarcoma. The atypia in the nuclei of the fat cells could be minimal. Marked variation in size of the fat cells is present. (H&E), original magnification 100x.

very poorly differentiated adipocytes) and interspersed lipoblasts (Fig. 3.21). Myxoid liposarcoma and round cell liposarcoma most commonly occur in the medial thigh and popliteal area. Myxoid liposarcoma is usually cured by surgical excision with or without adjuvant radiation therapy. The five-year survival rate for myxoid liposarcoma is about 90%. In contrast, round cell liposarcoma commonly metastasizes after excision with a five-year survival of only about 20% (11).

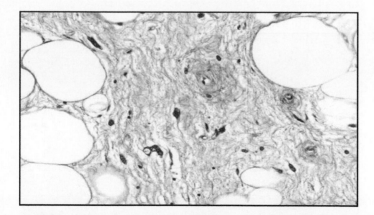

Figure 3.18 Well-differentiated liposarcoma. In the absence of atypia in the adipocytes, the atypical cells in the fibrous bands are a clue to the diagnosis. (H&E), original magnification 200x.

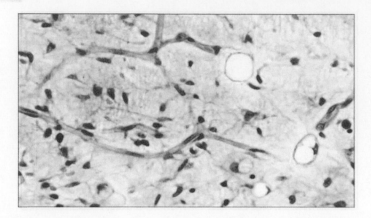

Figure 3.19   Myxoid liposarcoma: small, round to oval mesenchymal cells in a myxoid stroma with delicate arborizing blood vessels. (H&E), original magnification 400x.

Dedifferentiated liposarcoma is a malignant neoplasm composed of two clearly distinct cell types. There is an abrupt transition from well-differentiated liposarcoma to high-grade nonlipogenic sarcoma (Figs. 3.22 and 3.23). In about 90% of the cases, this pattern occurs in the primary tumor. The remaining 10% are seen in recurrent tumors, in which the primary tumor had been well-differentiated liposarcoma (12). Patients with dedifferentiated liposarcoma can be treated with surgical excision and postoperative chemotherapy.

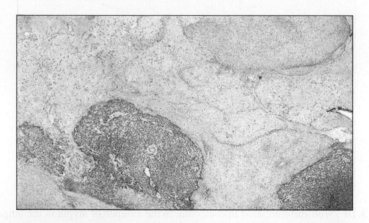

Figure 3.20   Myxoid liposarcoma with progression to round cell type (dark lobular areas). (H&E), original magnification 100x.

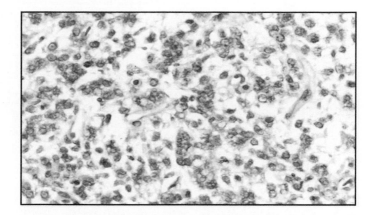

Figure 3.21 Round cell liposarcoma showing sheets of back-to-back small primitive cells with scant cytoplasm. (H&E), original magnification 200x.

Pleomorphic liposarcoma is the rarest subtype of liposarcoma and can easily be distinguished from other high-grade sarcomas by the presence of pleomorphic lipoblasts, and variably sized and shaped multinucleated cells (Fig. 3.24) (13). It tends to occur on the limbs of older adults, and may also be found on the trunk and retroperitoneum. This subtype is more aggressive than myxoid liposarcoma but less so than round cell liposarcoma, with a recurrence rate of 28%, metastatic rate of 44%, and mortality rate of 50% (12). Patients are

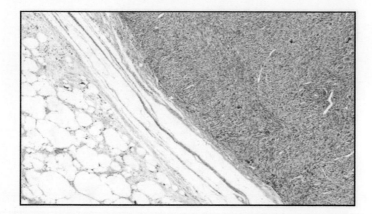

Figure 3.22 Dedifferentitated liposarcoma (upper right) arisen from a well-differentiated liposarcoma (lower left). There is a sharp demarcation between the two components. (H&E), original magnification 100x.

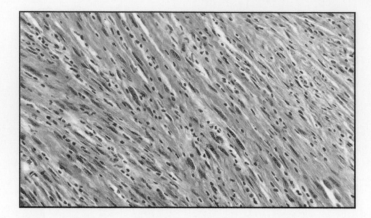

Figure 3.23   High-power view of dedifferentiated liposarcoma. Fascicles of spindle cells with atypical hyperchromatic nuclei are seen. (H&E), original magnification 200x.

often treated by surgical excision and postoperative radiation therapy. In some cases, chemotherapy may be added.

As the name implies, mixed-type liposarcomas show features of myxoid/ round cell, well-differentiated, dedifferentiated, and pleomorphic liposarcomas. These tumors are extremely rare and occur predominantly in elderly patients (2). Surgical excision and postoperative radiation therapy can be used to treat patients with mixed-type liposarcoma. Prognosis depends on the overall histological appearance, and also on the extent and location of the tumor.

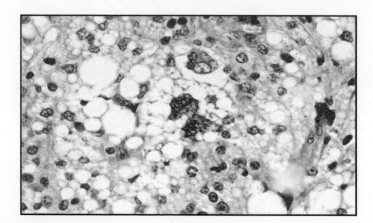

Figure 3.24   Pleomorphic liposarcoma: large cells with hyperchromatic and pleomorphic nuclei. A lipoblast with enlarged atypical nucleus scalloped by multiple cytoplasmic vacuoles is seen in the center. (H&E), original magnification 400x.

Finally, liposarcoma not otherwise specified is the category representing liposarcomas that histologically do not fit within the other categories discussed in the preceding sections.

STAGING OF LIPOSARCOMA

Accurate staging of liposarcoma is critical in determining a patient's diagnosis and selecting effective treatment options. A vast majority can be treated through surgical excision, either alone or in combination with radiation therapy. Adjuvant chemotherapy is used in selected patients. Liposarcoma does not have its own staging system but is staged according to soft tissue sarcoma staging systems, which are based on histological and clinical information. The most widely used staging system for soft tissue sarcomas is the American Joint Committee on Cancer (AJCC) and the Union for International Cancer Control (UICC) staging system. This system combines important determinants of survival in localized soft tissue sarcomas, such as the grade, depth of involvement, and size of tumor (14).

Tumor grades are based on summation scores assessing (*i*) differentiation, (*ii*) mitotic activity, and (*iii*) extent of necrosis.

Tumor differentiation is scored as follows:

- Score 1: sarcomas resembling normal, mature, mesenchymal tissues
- Score 2: sarcomas of definite histological type
- Score 3: synovial sarcomas, embryonal sarcomas, undifferentiated sarcomas, and sarcomas of unknown/doubtful tumor type

Mitotic count is assessed using 10 successive high-power fields (HPFs) in the most mitotically active area of the sarcoma (15). Mitotic count is scored as follows:

- Score 1: 0–9 mitoses per HPF
- Score 2: 10–19 mitoses per HPF
- Score 3: 20 or more mitoses per HPF

Tumor necrosis is evaluated by gross examination and validated by histological sections. Tumor necrosis is scored as follows:

- Score 0: no tumor necrosis
- Score 1: less than or equal to 50% tumor necrosis
- Score 2: more than 50% necrosis

Tumor grades are designated by summing the above scores as follows:

- Grade X (grade cannot be assessed)
- Grade 1 (total score 2 to 3)
- Grade 2 (total score 4 to 5)
- Grade 3 (total score 6 to 8)

Soft tissue sarcomas are divided by tumor size into two groups: T1 lesions are less than or equal to 5 cm, whereas T2 lesions are larger than 5 cm (15). Depth is evaluated in terms of the involvement of the adjacent fascia. Thus, tumors with no involvement of muscular fascia are categorized as superficial, or "a," tumors, whereas tumors with the involvement of muscular fascia are categorized as deep, or "b," tumors (15,16). The presence or absence of lymph node involvement is indicated by N1 and N0, respectively, whereas the presence or absence of metastases is indicated by M1 and M0, respectively.

Tumor stage is assigned by combining the information about tumor grade, size, and metastases. Stages I to III describe localized tumors, whereas stage IV applies to tumors that have metastasized to distant organs. Consequently, stages are designated as follows:

- Stage IA: grade 1 or X, less than 5 cm, no nodal or distant metastases
- Stage IB: same as 1A, but greater than 5 cm
- Stage IIA: grade 2 or 3, less than 5 cm, no nodal or distant metastases
- Stage IIB: same as IIA, but greater than 5 cm and grade 2 only
- Stage III: greater than 5cm and grade 3 *or* any size, any grade with nodal involvement but no distant metastases
- Stage IV: distant metastases

One limitation of the AJCC/UICC staging system is that it does not take into account the anatomic location of the tumor, which can be an important determinant of patient treatment and outcome (2). However, the five-year survival rates for stages I, II, III, and IV are 90%, 70%, 50%, and 10% to 20%, respectively, indicating that the staging system is effective in establishing prognostic breakpoints (16,17). A more important limitation is that liposarcoma is grouped in this staging system with other, possibly more aggressive, soft tissue sarcomas and the prognostic accuracy of the staging system for liposarcoma has not been well established. Given the rarity of liposarcoma, it would be difficult to accumulate enough data to develop a unique staging system for this disease. Nonetheless, it is important to have such reproducible and uniform staging criteria to allow comparison of clinical experiences among cancer centers and for determining clinical trial eligibility (16).

CONCLUSION

Adipocytic tumors are diverse neoplasms that have a spectrum of clinical manifestations, treatment options, and prognosis. Although lipomas are common and easily diagnosed clinically, clinicians should have an increased suspicion when evaluating larger subcutaneous tumors, rapidly appearing or growing lesions, deeper tumors with possible extension beyond the subcutaneous fat, and symptomatic tumors, such as in lipomatosis of nerve. Radiological imaging and biopsy prior to definitive surgical excision may be considered in such cases. Liposarcoma may be suspected in large or growing lesions. In such cases, rapid diagnosis is critical, since tumor size is a major risk factor for recurrence and death. Surgery is the primary form of treatment and is curative for most adipocytic tumors. Radiation therapy can be effective in selected cases. Chemotherapy has little to no effect on most liposarcomas. Future studies investigating the molecular and genetic pathogenesis of these tumors will be valuable in improving patient outcomes.

REFERENCES

1. Levy-Marchal C, Pénicaud L. Adipose Tissue Development: From Animal Models to Clinical Conditions. Switzerland: Karger, 2010.
2. Fletcher C, Unni K, Mertens F, eds. Pathology and Genetics: Tumors of Soft Tissue and Bone. Lyon: IARC Press, 2002.
3. Bancroft L, Kransdorf M, Peterson J, et al. Benign fatty tumors: classification, clinical course, imaging appearance, and treatment. Skeletal Radiol 2006; 35: 719–733.
4. Hameed M. Pathology and genetics of adipocytic tumors. Cytogenet Genome Res 2007; 118:138–147.
5. Enzinger F, Weiss S. Soft Tissue Tumors. St. Louis: Mosby, 2001.
6. Murphey M, Carroll J, Felmming D, et al. From the archives of the AFIP: benign musculoskeletal lipomatous lesions. Radiographics 2004; 24:1433–1466.
7. Chung E, Enzinger F. Benign lipoblastomatosis: an analysis of 35 cases. Cancer 1973; 32:482–492.
8. Prahlow J. Extra-adrenal myelolipoma: report of two cases. South Med J 1995; 88:639.
9. Heinz-Peer G. Abdomen: retroperitoneum, adrenals, kidney and upper urinary tract. In: Reimer P, Parizel P, Meaney J, eds. Clinical MR Imaging: A Practical Approach. 3rd ed. New York: Springer, 2010:430–431.
10. Kransdorf M, Murphey M. Imaging of Soft Tissue Tumors. Philadelphia: Lippincott Williams & Wilkins, 2006.
11. Åkerman M, Domanski H. The Cytology of Soft Tissue Tumors. Switzerland: Karger, 2003.
12. Dei Tos A. Liposarcoma: new entities and evolving concepts. Ann Diagn Pathol 2000; 4:252–266.
13. Downes K, Goldblum J, Montgomery A, et al. Pleomorphic liposarcoma: a clinicopathologic examination of 19 cases. Mod Pathol 2001; 14:179–184.
14. Clark M, Fisher C, Judson I, et al. Soft tissue sarcomas in adults. N Engl J Med 2005; 353:701–711.
15. American Joint Committee on Cancer (AJCC). Soft tissue sarcoma. In: Edge S, Byrd D, Compton C, eds. Cancer Staging Manual. 7th ed. New York: Springer, 2010: 291–298.
16. Cormier J, Pollock R. Soft tissue sarcomas. Cancer 2004; 54:94–109.
17. Stojadinovic A, Leung D, Allen P, et al. Primary adult soft tissue sarcoma: time dependent influence of prognostic variables. J Clin Oncol 2002; 20:4344–4352.

4

Liposuction

Jason Marquart and Naomi Lawrence

INTRODUCTION

Modern liposuction is the art of contouring of the body through removal of adipose tissue using mechanical suction techniques. This chapter reviews the history of liposuction, safety, preoperative preparation, procedure sequence, and advanced techniques. Following review of this information, the reader will gain the knowledge to develop skills in the technique of the procedure and be able to successfully adapt them to clinical practice.

BACKGROUND

Lipocontouring has evolved dramatically over the last century (Table 4.1). In its beginnings, it involved manual extirpation of fat through skin incisions and excision of overlying redundant skin (1,2). The procedure then evolved to a suction-based technique. The next major advance was the development of the blunt cannula, which was used to methodically and less traumatically extract the fat through intersecting tunnels (3,4).

Suction-based fat removal developed along the lines of manual and mechanical techniques. The manual suction technique was popularized by Fournier, particularly because of his interest in fat transfer (5). On the other hand, the mechanical technique evolved from the use of a suction device developed for gynecologic procedures. Illouz, who pioneered this technique, was also credited with development of the technique of tumescing the treatment area prior to suction (6). This "wet technique" utilized hypotonic saline and hyaluronidase, which he believed would enhance lipolysis (6,7). In contrast, the "dry technique" involves suction of the fat while the patient is under general anesthesia without tumescence of the treatment area.

The next major milestone in liposuction was the development of tumescent anesthesia, further advancing the "wet technique" by creating profound local anesthesia and thus allowing the procedure to be done without the use of general sedation (8). The safety of this anesthetic technique was validated by Klein as well as others (9–12). Besides the obvious benefits from enhanced safety, tumescent liposuction allows the removal of significant amounts of adipose tissue with excellent contour correction and minimal postoperative morbidity.

Table 4.1 Historical Timeline

1921: Dujarrier (France) uses a uterine curette to remove fat from a ballerina's knees, which ultimately resulted in loss of the patient's legs because of gangrene (2,13).

1960s: Josef Schrudde (Germany) introduces suction removal of fat following sharp curettage of the hips, thighs, knees, and ankles (2).

1970s: Kesselring and Meyer (Switzerland) introduce suction fat curettage (14).

Mid-1970s: Georgio Fischer and Arpad Fischer (Italy) introduce the idea of fat removal through subcutaneous blunt cannulas (3,4).

Early 1980s: Richard Webster and Julius Newman of the American Academy of Cosmetic Surgery found the American Society of Liposuction Surgery and develop training courses to teach the technique (15).

Early 1980s: Fournier and Illouz use a suction cannula as opposed to sharp curette; the former also recommends syringe-based suction and cross-tunneling (5,6).

1982: Illouz, father of modern liposuction, introduces "suction-assisted lipolysis" and "wet" liposuction with infusion of saline in the target area prior to the procedure (5).

1985: Jeffrey Klein, an American dermatologic surgeon, revolutionizes liposuction with the development of tumescent anesthesia, allowing safe, in-office removal of large volumes of fat with negligible blood loss, quick patient recovery, and excellent cosmetic results. Klein published two key scientific studies detailing the pharmacology of tumescent lidocaine anesthesia and tumescent technique (8,9).

Late 1980s: American surgeons begin learning and developing the technique in the United States. At the same time, liposuction training is introduced into Dermatology residency programs.

1987: The American Academy of Dermatology adds liposuction to the core surgical curriculum for dermatology residents (16).

1989: The American Academy of Dermatology is the first medical specialty group to develop liposuction guidelines (16).

1996 and 1998: Klochn and Zocchi introduce ultrasound-assisted liposuction (17–19).

2000s: Laser-assisted liposuction is introduced (20).

CURRENT STATE OF KNOWLEDGE

Procedure Overview

Tumescent liposuction combines regional anesthesia with subcutaneous fat removal. This anesthetic technique utilizes large volumes of dilute lidocaine and epinephrine, which are infused into the subcutaneous space to provide significant localized anesthesia, and obviates the earlier requirements for general anesthesia. Since only local anesthesia is used, together with minimal adjunctive sedation or pain medication, the safety profile is dramatically improved (21).

The pharmacokinetics of the tumescent anesthetic solution is significantly different from that of the 1% lidocaine solution, which allows for large volumes to be safely infused with minimal systemic effects. The dilute—0.05% to 0.1%—lidocaine mixed with 1:1,000,000 to 1:2,000,000 concentration of epinephrine reduces, as well as delays by 4 to 14 hours, the peak serum levels of the anesthetic (8,12). This is in contrast with the standard 1% lidocaine solution, which results in higher peak levels, typically reached in 15 to 30 minutes (22,23). Thus, the maximum recommended safe dose of lidocaine for local, nontumescent anesthesia ranges from 35 to 55 mg/kg, depending on the concomitant use of medications that affect lidocaine metabolism through their interaction with the cytochrome P450 system (Table 4.2) (12,24–26).

Following the infusion of the anesthetic solution into the targeted treatment areas, the adipose tissue is suctioned out through small cannulas that are inserted through the infusion ports. Additional suction ports through the skin may be needed to reach all parts of the treatment area because of the variability in patient contour or anatomy. The aspirate consists of a mixture of fat, tumescent solution, and blood, with the latter component being significantly smaller compared with that in the "dry" method of liposuction (27).

Safety

The safety of tumescent liposuction has been extensively validated since its inception in the late 1980s. In fact, it is the safest way to provide correction in body contour through the removal of adipose tissue. When compared with nontumescent liposuction, the risk of fatality is extremely low. Furthermore, the current data support its safety as an office-based, as opposed to hospital-based, procedure. Most of the risks of serious adverse events and mortality from liposuction are related to general anesthesia (Table 4.3).

Training

The suggested sequence of training to gain the skill set necessary to perform liposuction should include several components (35,36). These consist of residency training and board certification in an appropriate field that receives instruction in cutaneous surgery, such as dermatology or plastic surgery, training in liposuction techniques during residency or fellowship or through an appropriate liposuction course that includes didactic and "hands-on" training by a physician experienced in the technique, and live surgical exercises with active participation. In addition, the trainee should gain knowledge in preparation of the tumescent anesthetic and anesthetic infusion techniques, cannula and equipment

Table 4.2 Common Drug Interactions with Lidocaine

Antimicrobials
   Antibiotics
      Ciprofloxacin
      Clarithromycin
      Erythromycin
      Norfloxacin
      Sparfloxacin
   Antifungals
      Fluconazole
      Ketoconazole
      Itraconazole
Antidepressants
   Selective serotonin reuptake inhibitors
      Citalopram
      Fluoxetine
      Fluvoxamine
      Norfluoxetine
      Paroxetine
      Sertraline
   Other antidepressants
      Nefazodone
Calcium-channel blockers
   Diltiazem
   Nifedipine
   Verapamil
Other inhibitors
   Bromocriptine
   Cimetidine
   Cyclosporine
   Grapefruit juice
   Methadone
   Methlyprednisolone
   Tamoxifen
   Valproic acid
   Zafirlukast

choices, and management of complications such as fluid and electrolyte imbalances and lidocaine toxicity. Furthermore, trainees should be proctored by a qualified instructor on the first 5 to 10 liposuction cases until an appropriate level of competence is verified and a log of liposuction procedures should be maintained. Physicians planning to perform tumescent liposuction should have current Basic Life Support and Advanced Cardiac Life Support certifications.

Table 4.3 Studies on Tumescent Liposuction Safety

1988 (Hanke et al.): Survey of 55 dermatologists and 9478 liposuction cases. Systemic
   complication risk was 0.07%. 5 cases developed "excessive" intraoperative or
   postoperative blood loss, and 2 cases had infection. No cases of disseminated
   intravascular coagulation, fat emboli, perforated viscus, thrombophlebitis, or death.
   Low risk of local complications, including postoperative contour irregularities (2.1%),
   hematoma (0.47%), and persistent postoperative edema (0.46%) (28).
1996 (Hanke et al.): Survey of the American Society for Dermatologic Surgery fellows,
   15,336 liposuction cases. No serious complications reported (29).
1999 (Coleman et al.): Analysis of the National Database of the Physicians Insurance
   Association of America on malpractice data (199–1997), evaluating the effect of the
   location of the liposuction procedure and physician specialty on the incidence of
   malpractice claims. Hospital-based liposuction had triple the amount of malpractice
   settlements as opposed to office-based liposuction. Of the defendants, 90% were
   plastic surgeons and less than 1% were dermasurgeons (30).
2002 (Housman et al.): National survey of more than 66,570 liposuction cases. No
   reported deaths; serious adverse event rate was 0.68 per 1000 cases. 74% of cases were
   performed in office (31).
2002 (Coldiron et al.): Review of Florida adverse event data. No tumescent anesthesia-
   related liposuction deaths were reported; 2 deaths were related to liposuction under
   general anesthesia (32).
2004 (Coldiron et al.): Review of Florida adverse event data from 2000 to 2003. Again, no
   tumescent anesthesia-related liposuction deaths were reported, while 2 deaths were
   related to liposuction under general anesthesia (33).
2007 (Coldiron et al.): Review of Florida adverse event data 2002–2007. No tumescent
   anesthesia-related liposuction deaths were seen, while 8 deaths were related to
   liposuction under general anesthesia (34).

Indications

Tumescent liposuction serves primarily as a method of aesthetic body contouring, but may also be used for several medical conditions, including lipomas,
axillary hyperhidrosis and bromhidrosis, gynecomastia, lipodystrophy, and
thinning of flaps and scars (Table 4.4). Cosmetic applications of liposuction
involve the reduction of adipose pockets that are resistant to dietary modifications and exercise. Examples of locations that may benefit from this procedure include the neck, arms, breasts, abdomen, back, flanks, buttocks, hips,
thighs, and knees (21,35,36).

   Patient selection is a key factor to the success of a liposuction procedure
(Table 4.5). Patients at their ideal body weight or within 20% above their ideal
body weight may consider liposuction as a means of improving their general
body contour and to achieve a better fit for their clothing. Liposuction should
not, however, be employed for weight loss. Thus, if a patient is morbidly obese,

Table 4.4 Liposuction Indications

Contour pockets of adiposity in patients near their ideal body weight with disproportional deposits

Aesthetic contouring
    Face: jowls, buccal, and lateral nasolabial
    Neck: submental and lateral
    Torso: breasts, abdomen, flanks, back, and hips
    Extremities: arms, buttocks, thighs, knees, calves, and ankles

Medical
    Lipomas
    Axillary hyperhidrosis and bromhidrosis
    Gynecomastia
    Lipodystrophy (HIV, Cushing Syndrome)
    Evacuation of hematomas and seromas
    Lymphedema

Reconstruction
    Flap movement/elevation
    Fat debulking following flap or graft

Source: From Refs. 21, 35, and 36.

bariatric surgery (gastric bypass or lapbanding) may be the recommended treatment course. Also, if weight loss is the patient's primary goal for the procedure, a weight loss program with focus on behavior modification may be a better therapeutic option. Nonetheless, liposuction may have a secondary benefit of motivating a patient to begin an exercise and dietary modification program, which then contributes to the overall success of the procedure.

The best candidate has a relatively stable ideal body weight, which has been maintained over the previous 6 to 12 months. On the other hand, a patient who does not have a stable weight is at an increased risk for weight gain and subsequent loss of benefits following the procedure. Moreover, in cases of weight gain following fat removal by liposuction, the newly accumulated fat tends to deposit in inaccessible locations. For example, fat removed via liposuction from the subcutaneous plane of the abdomen tends to instead be deposited deep to the rectus abdominis muscle and around the viscera.

Preoperative Preparation

A comprehensive yet focused evaluation of the liposuction candidate should be conducted preoperatively (37). An effective office consultation can take up to an hour of office resources, but can be weighted toward the cosmetic consultant. The primary objective of the office consultation is to identify the appropriate candidate. A preconsultation questionnaire is a useful tool, which

Table 4.5 Liposuction Contraindications

Absolute
    Pregnancy
    Eating disorders (anorexia nervosa or bulimia) and body dysmorphic disorder by
        DSM-IV criteria
    Hematologic: uncorrectable abnormalities or anticoagulant requirements
    Abdominal hernia
    Lidocaine allergy
    Pulmonary embolism
    Thrombophlebitis
Relative
    Cellulite
    Weight loss or obesity (experimental)
Caution
    Unrealistic expectations
    Weight instability, recent significant weight loss, or difficulty maintaining current
        weight
    Very-low-calorie diet
Medical clearance required
    Cardiac disease
    Diabetes
    Hypertension
    Liver disease
    Immunosuppression
    Hypercoagulability, including history of thromboembolism or deep vein thrombosis,
        factor V Leiden, protein C or S deficiency, lupus anticoagulant, smoking, high-
        dose estrogen

can provide a wealth of information and quickly exclude poor surgical candidates. Information that should be sought through the questionnaire and subsequent consultation includes weight control issues, methods of dieting, physical activity, genetic components of body shape, and location of desired treatment areas. Particular attention should be paid to unusual requests, unrealistic expectations, and other criteria indicative of a body dysmorphic disorder. Concerns and contraindications to surgery should also be addressed. The liposuction procedure should be thoroughly discussed with an emphasis on risks, benefits, realistic outcomes, and the possibility of a repeat procedure for unresponsive areas. It should also be stressed that although liposuction can quickly alter body contour by removing fat, the maximal benefits are typically not obtained for several months pending the retraction of redundant skin.

    Once the medical component of the consultation is completed and the patient is deemed a potential candidate for the procedure, pricing is reviewed with the cosmetic consultant. Pricing is typically given for the treatment of bilateral regions, such as both flanks, outer thighs, and so forth. The size of the treatment area also influences the quoted price, since larger areas require longer time to infuse the tumescent anesthesia and longer suctioning time, resulting in increased cost to the provider. In addition, the size of the area and the number of treatment locations are important, since the procedure is limited by the maximum dose of tumescent anesthesia and may require partitioning into two or more sessions.

Medical and Surgical History

As with all elective cosmetic procedures, the risks should be weighed against the benefits. Screening candidates for medical conditions that increase the potential for adverse outcomes should be a primary focus. Patients in higher-risk categories because of age (older than 60 years), diabetes, hypertension, cardiac history, immunosuppression, and other significant medical history should be referred for medical clearance (37). Immunosuppression from diabetes, HIV, and medications increases the risk of infection. Liver dysfunction from alcohol-induced or infectious hepatitis, chemotherapy, and highly active antiretroviral therapy may increase the potential for lidocaine toxicity (38–40). Surgery increases the risk of deep vein thrombosis and thromboembolic events, effects that can be further compounded in patients with hypercoagulable states such as smokers, those taking high-dose estrogen, or those with protein C/S deficiency or with malignancy (41). On the other hand, a history of prolonged bleeding from various disorders may be difficult to assess from laboratory tests such as coagulation studies and platelet counts. Thus, the patient needs to be carefully questioned about prolonged bleeding from prior procedures and, if a bleeding disorder is suspected, may require evaluation by a hematologist prior to proceeding.

Prior surgical history should focus on procedures in the area of liposuction, which can limit the ability to move the cannula because of scar tissue. Previous liposuction in the treatment area can also limit the amount of fat return because of the fibrous nature of the remaining fat. It can also cause increased pain with tumescent anesthesia infusion. The physician should also take extreme care when evaluating previously treated areas to ensure that the location of fat is accessible. A patient with a history of abdominal surgery should be carefully questioned about dehiscences or infections and examined for evidence of hernia, which may create a void in the rectus muscle and expose the abdominal viscera to trauma from the cannula. If there is a concern for communication with the internal abdominal cavity, a thorough evaluation with imaging, as well as communication with the patient's surgeon should be conducted. The patient should also be examined for keloids or hypertrophic scars and, if present, a risk of unsightly scarring at the incision sites should be discussed.

Table 4.6 Preoperative Laboratory Studies

Urine pregnancy test (obtained on the day of surgery)
Cell blood count (CBC) with differential
General chemistry panel
Prothrombin and partial thromboplastin time (PT/PTT)
Hepatitis panel
HIV antibodies

Laboratory Studies

Laboratory tests are recommended for all patients undergoing larger-volume liposuction (>250 cc) because of the increased risk of lidocaine toxicity (Table 4.6). It is recommended that a urine pregnancy test in all women of childbearing potential be performed on the day of the procedure. Some institutions may also require screening for infectious diseases, such as hepatitis B and C and HIV in any patient undergoing surgical treatment (21,35,36).

Medical Allergies

The patient should be queried about all allergies with the exception of seasonal allergic rhinitis. There are multiple facets to the procedure that can put the patient at risk for an allergic reaction. A history of allergy to medications, latex, and contactants (surgical scrub, adhesives, etc.) needs to be thoroughly evaluated. Focus should be placed on anaphylactic and systemic reactions, but contact dermatitis can sometimes be equally problematic. Tumescent solutions typically contain a mixture of lidocaine, epinephrine, and bicarbonate in normal saline. Although uncommon, each component, as well as its preservative, can cause allergic reactions. Most allergies ascribed to the lidocaine mixture are actually to the preservative methyl paraben. This issue can be easily remedied by using a preservative-free formulation. It should be noted that this allergen has the potential to cross-react with para-aminobenzoic acid (PABA), which is a metabolite of ester anesthetics, which should then also be avoided (42). A true allergy to lidocaine is extremely rare and is an absolute contraindication to the procedure. Other anesthetics, such as prilocaine, have also been tried; however, there is an increased risk of toxicity from such agents. A consultation with an allergist for provocative testing may be necessary. Although allergies to epinephrine do not exist, since it is a natural component of the endocrine system, reactions to the epinephrine solution may be due to preservatives or to the agent's sympathomimetic effects. Symptoms of tachycardia, preventricular contractions, and shaking ("jitteriness") are often confused with allergy but are more consistent with sensitivity to catecholamines (22). Given the low dilution of epinephrine (0.65 mg of 1:1000) in tumescent solution and the low vascularity of adipose tissue, tachycardia is rare. If encountered, tachycardia can be easily remedied in normotensive patients with 0.1 mg of clonidine.

Antistaphylococcal antibiotics are typically prescribed preoperatively and commonly require modifications because of patient allergies. In our practice, cefazolin is used intravenously 30 minutes prior to the procedure. If a patient has an allergy to cephalosporins or penicillins, oral clindamycin is given the night prior to and 30 minutes before surgery. Given the high incidence of methicillin-resistant *Staphylococcus aureus* and inducible clindamycin resistance in certain populations, trimethoprim-sulfamethoxazole may become an increasingly utilized alternative in nonsulfa allergic patients. However, in such cases, the maximum dose of lidocaine may need to be decreased because of the agent's interaction with cytochrome p450. Other medications that are sometimes used during the procedure include lorazepam and fentanyl for their anxiolytic and sedative properties. Allergies to these classes of drugs may necessitate substitutions such as diazepam, which may subsequently require a decrease in the maximum lidocaine dose.

Latex allergies and sensitivity should prompt utilization of latex-free gloves, garments, tubes, and dressings to avoid systemic anaphylactic reactions. Contact allergy to skin preparation agents such as iodine, hexachlorophene, and chlorhexidine is another potential issue that may need to be addressed. Patients may also describe sensitivity to adhesives from bandages, which should prompt a substitution with hypoallergic adhesives, as in paper tape.

Medication History

A thorough list of medications should include all agents consumed by the patient, such as prescriptions, herbal supplements, vitamins, hormones, and over-the-counter products. The patient should also be asked about medications and supplements with anticoagulant effects. If possible, anticoagulant agents should be discontinued according to the number of days required for their effect to dissipate (Table 4.7) (43); if they cannot be stopped for medical reasons,

Table 4.7 Anticoagulant Effects of Nonsteroidal Anti-inflammatory Agents

NSAID	Half-Life (Hours)	Preoperative Management
Aspirin[a]	0.25–0.3	Hold 10–14 days prior to surgery
Naproxen	12–15	Hold 4 days prior to surgery
Ibuprofen	1.8–2	Hold 1 day prior to surgery
Diclofenac	2	Hold 1 day prior to surgery
Indomethacin	4.5	Hold 1 day prior to surgery
Nabumetone	23–24	Hold 5 days prior to surgery
Piroxicam	50	Hold 10 days prior to surgery

[a]Despite the short half-life of aspirin, platelets are irreversibly inhibited and require 10–14 days to regenerate. *Source*: From Ref. 43.

liposuction is contraindicated. For example, patients who require warfarin or clopidogrel are likely noncandidates for liposuction because of significant medical issues that necessitated these agents in the first place. It is recommended that all herbal supplements be discontinued prior to surgery because of potential anticoagulant effects. Some common supplements that may significantly affect coagulation—particularly when used with other anticoagulants—include bilberry, chondroitin, Dong Quai root, feverfew, garlic, ginger, ginkgo, ginseng, and vitamin E (44).

Hormonal therapy with estrogen may enhance the risk of thrombosis. Low-dose oral contraceptives are considered to pose little risk (45). In contrast, high-dose estrogen-containing hormonal replacement therapy in combination with smoking dramatically increases the risk of thromboembolism, especially in the first year of therapy (46–49). In such cases, hormone cessation is recommended to reduce the risk of adverse events.

Medications should be assessed for their effect on the hepatic cytochrome p450 system, which is the primary route of lidocaine metabolism (Table 4.2). If a medication is noted to have an inhibitory effect on this system, its use should be avoided prior to surgery with enough time to dissipate, as determined by its half-life. As an example, selective serotonin inhibitors may require several weeks to clear from the body. If an inhibitory agent cannot be stopped, the maximum lidocaine dose should be decreased to 35 mg/kg.

Weight and Fitness

The total number of fat cells increases through adulthood and stabilizes around a genetically determined set point. Obese patients tend to add more fat cells per year than thinner patients. Liposuction is a means of providing short-term benefits by reducing the volume of adipose tissue. It also transiently reduces the total number of adipocytes; however, these cells are replaced by stem cells to maintain homeostasis around the set point (50). To maintain the long-term benefits of liposuction, a comprehensive evaluation of the patient's weight trends is essential and allows the physician to predict patient's ability to retain the benefits of contour enhancement following the procedure. Many individuals continually trend up and down around a certain weight set point. In individuals who use dieting as a primary means of maintaining weight as opposed to exercise or a combination of diet and exercise, weight regain is significantly higher (51–53). People who exercise and diet lose the most weight; however, people who exercise alone are more apt to maintain the weight loss (53).

The type of diet also has a significant impact on the ability to maintain weight loss. The most successful diets combine behavior modification with increased protein and decreased carbohydrate intake (54). This formula improves the patient's ability to moderate caloric intake and directs the body to burn fat as opposed to carbohydrates, which increases the overall caloric expenditure (55–58). In contrast, very-low-calorie and low-fat diets cause the body to shift into a metabolic starvation mode. The body's metabolism subsequently decreases to conserve energy and protein is burned instead of fat, resulting in loss of muscle mass. Furthermore, such dieters tend to remain continuously hungry and are more likely to develop binge-eating behavior (55).

Exercise can significantly impact maintenance of weight by increasing the basal metabolic rate (59). It improves muscle tone and maximizes the contour of the area prior to removing excess adiposity. In females, muscle tone can significantly affect treatment recommendations for certain areas such as the abdomen and arms.

In the abdomen, the contour abnormality may be related to a combination of poor muscle tone, subcutaneous adiposity, and visceral adiposity. A proper assessment of each of these abdominal components will provide the patient with the appropriate sequence to improvement. A lax rectus requires an increase in weight-bearing exercise, as opposed to visceral fat, which requires a combination of exercise and dieting. For patients with subcutaneous deposits of fat recalcitrant to diet and exercise, liposuction would be a potential option.

The upper arms may also have a combination of inadequate muscle tone, redundant skin, and adiposity that creates a less desirable appearance. To properly address this area, all three features must be assessed. In patients with poor muscle tone and limited adiposity, an increase in weight-bearing exercise is recommended. In patients with good muscle tone with areas of adiposity, liposuction may be of benefit. Laxity of skin, which can limit the amount of correction in the contour, should also be assessed. Patients with lax skin tend to retract less than patients with good elasticity, which may result in a suboptimal correction despite removal of equivalent amounts of fat. These patients should be thus counseled and surgical removal of redundant skin should be mentioned as a possible treatment option. However, the amount of scarring involved with this type of correction needs to be discussed.

Expectations

As with any cosmetic procedure, realistic, achievable patient goals should be assessed. Overall, most patients have realistic expectations of what liposuction can achieve (60). Preoperative screening through the use of a questionnaire and dialogue help to detect patients with unreasonable goals. For example, patients who believe that liposuction is primarily a means for weight loss should be thoroughly educated about the true purpose of the procedure: creation of a more aesthetic appearance by contouring disproportionate areas of adiposity.

Ideal candidates are at their ideal body weight or moderately overweight with moderate areas of accessible adipose deposits. Such patients will often gain additional motivation to increase their exercise and improve their diet following the procedure. In contrast, morbidly obese patients may not benefit as significantly from liposuction, as smaller proportion of fat will be removed relative to the overall body fat, which translates to a less noticeable contour correction.

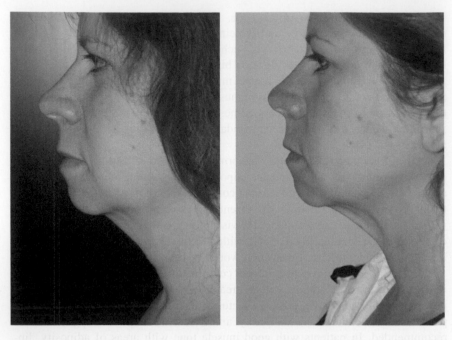

Figure 4.1 Pre (*left*) and post (*right*) submental liposuction. Patient was dissatisfied with the results because of residual skin redundancy, which she felt precluded her from wearing a tight necklace.

Careful attention should be paid to specific comments made by a potential candidate regarding his or her expectations from the procedure. Open-ended questions are most helpful in this situation, such as "What do you plan to achieve from the liposuction procedure?" As an example, a patient in our practice desired to be able to wear a "choker" necklace following a submental liposuction procedure but was unable to achieve this goal despite improved contour (Fig. 4.1). Consequently, she was dissatisfied with the procedure results. This situation could have been prevented by inquiring about patient's specific goals and explaining that skin texture and quality might preclude wearing a tight necklace, even with an improved contour.

By properly examining the patient's muscle tone, skin laxity, bone structure, and fat compartment localization, the physician can provide more insight into the patient's anatomy and create a more accurate understanding of the anticipated end result following the procedure. This also opens a dialogue on alternate procedures that may further benefit the patient. Although the patient may still desire to proceed with liposuction despite its potential limitations, proper preoperative counseling is more likely to lead to an acceptance of suboptimal outcomes as dictated by his or her unique anatomy.

Table 4.8 Physical Examination

Body contour (may be a source of body fullness not amenable to liposuction)
Asymmetry (scoliosis, muscle bulk)
Pelvis shape (gynecoid or android)
Neck (anterior hyoid, thyroid, glandular)
Muscle bulk (arms, back, buttocks, anterior thighs, and calves)
Muscle tone (poor abdominal and brachial tone may be an important contributor to
   contour as opposed to fat)

Physical Examination

Physical examination should focus on areas of adiposity amenable to liposuction, skin quality, asymmetry, and general health status for surgery (Table 4.8). Patients are examined while in a gown and in the upright position. Assessment of adipose deposits can be completed by visual inspection and tactile manipulation. With the latter techniques, pockets of fat are compressed with the palm of the hand or by grasping the skin and the underlying fat between the thumb and the index finger (Fig. 4.2). These assessments can be facilitated by correct patient positioning and contraction of the underlying musculature. Regional locations of fat deposits should be described and diagrammed as specifically as possible— upper arms, abdomen (upper and lower), back, hips and waist, thighs (inner and outer), knees, and others (Table 4.9)—as these have a direct bearing on the specific techniques utilized at every stage of the procedure (Table 4.10). In patients with multiple areas of adiposity, regional treatments should be recommended to prevent relative accentuation of adjacent untreated locations. Thus,

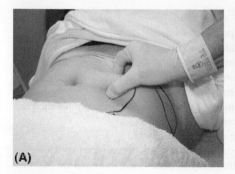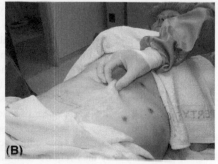

(A)   **(B)**

Figure 4.2 Pinch test: **(A)** preprocedure and **(B)** postprocedure. Note the interval decrease in the thickness of skin pinch following the removal of adipose tissue.

Table 4.9 Regional Considerations

Neck (chin, cheek, jowls)
Assessment:
    Contract platysma (clench teeth) to enhance preplatysmal fat assessment and to assess for platysmal banding (plication may benefit) (61)
    Palpate hyoid to assess for anterior placement, which may limit attainable cosmetic result by making the neck angle appear more oblique
    Other causes of skin redundancy and fullness: enlarged thyroid, lymph nodes, submandibular salivary glands (62), and micrognathia
Best candidate: good elasticity, palpable submental fat pads, normal hyoid placement, absence of platysmal bands
    May require a combination of procedures such as plication (platysma and/or subcutaneous musculoaponeurotic system, implants, face-lift, and resurfacing); inelastic skin may increase vertical lines when fat is removed
Counseling: emphasize that contour irregularities and firmness are not uncommon for several months; males have a slower and decreased amount of retraction compared with females (62–64)

Arms (65)
Assessment: patient abducts arms to 90° and arm musculature and adiposity is palpated with contraction
Best candidate: primarily women with good elasticity, minimal laxity, and with adipose deposits in proximal arm noted with arm abduction
Counseling: skin redundancy may be significant and may remain despite removal of adipose tissue; patients should be advised that overall circumference will be improved but may be limited because of redundancy

Abdomen
Assessment: patient bends forward toward the toes in lateral hip-flexion, pinch test, muscle contraction to assess for subcutaneous versus visceral fat
Best candidate: young age, adequate elasticity, adiposity below umbilicus, and toned rectus
Subtypes (66)
    Lower abdomen
        Thin individual near the ideal body weight with lower abdomen deposits
        Excellent result potential and high patient satisfaction
        Also requires treatment of upper abdomen to maintain symmetry
    Upper and lower abdomen and back, posterior waist, and hips (female)
        Perimenopausal, older women on hormone replacement or following weight gain
    Upper and lower abdomen and flanks (male)
        Careful attention required in assessment of adipose location, since most men are noncandidates because of visceral location
    Lax abdomen postpregnancy or because of weight cycling
        Usually benefit from procedure because of retraction over several months
        Minority may also require abdominoplasty if there is lax skin and no residual fat; reassess in a few months postprocedure (65)

(Continued)

Breast (female) (67–70)

Assessment:

An expanded history with focus on history of breast cancer (family or personal)

All patients should receive a pre- and postoperative (6 months) mammogram; if preoperative abnormalities exist, the procedure should be deferred until the areas are properly evaluated

The breast should be measured preoperative with circumference and breast mass or volume

Best candidate: moderate breast size to avoid suboptimal outcomes such as nipple ptosis and excess skin redundancy, which requires surgical correction

Counseling: Repeat procedures may be needed to avoid removing excess volume (approximately one-third is adequate to start) and patient should be advised that a realistic reduction is by one cup size

Breast (male)

Assessment:

An expanded history assessing possible causes for gynecomastia (65)

Medications (clomiphene, diazepam, digoxin, phenytoin, spironolactone)

Endocrine tumors (testicular, pituitary, adrenal)

Hypogonadism

Alcoholism

Genetic adipose or glandular deposition

Palpation of the breast tissue with assessment of asymmetry and irregular, firm, fixed masses with appropriate imaging for abnormalities, as indicated (71)

Possible palpation of testes to assess for hormone-secreting tumors (71)

Best candidate: male with adipose deposition not related to external factors, good laxity

Counseling: will not completely remove adipose tissue and a conservative improvement is seen in approximately 50% (65); patients should be advised that glandular tissue may contribute to a suboptimal outcome and ultimately require excisional removal (71,72)

Knees and medial thighs

Assessment

Knee: fullness of this area is often due to a descent of the thigh. Therefore, if a contributor, the thigh should be considered for treatment

Medial thigh: assess anterior and posterior thigh to ensure proportions are maintained; avoid complete circumferential liposuction in a single procedure because of a risk of lymphostasis (65)

Best candidate: Well-localized adiposity, good elasticity and skin tone, and near ideal body weight.

Counseling: the medial thigh skin does not retract well and may result in a suboptimal outcome because of residual redundancy; avoid oversuctioning of knee. This may damage vasculature and lymphatics, which increases the risk of hematomas, seromas, and persistent hyperpigmentation (65)

(Continued)

Table 4.9 Regional Considerations (*Continued*)

Hips, outer thighs, and buttocks
Assessment
Outer thigh: patient contracts the gluteus maximus to observe the outer thigh contour. If the contour improves with contraction, buttocks contribute to the adipose pocket and the outer lower aspect of the buttocks should be considered for suctioning (73)
Best candidate: females with "saddlebag" deposition, good elasticity, and absence of cellulite.
Counseling: Be sure to note cellulite, poor skin elasticity, adiposity within the infragluteal fold, and muscular prominence, as these conditions cannot be enhanced with liposuction

the upper and lower abdomen or the hips/waist and outer thighs should be treated simultaneously.

Aspects of skin quality that may adversely affect retraction and remodeling include poor elasticity and tone and actinic damage (38). Elasticity and tone can be assessed by pinching the skin away from the body and releasing. Skin with good elasticity should recoil immediately in contrast to inelastic skin, which has a delayed return to its original position and may even have memory of the stretched position for several seconds. Patients with poor elasticity should be counseled on the possibility of residual redundant skin following the removal of subcutaneous fat, particularly in areas such as the upper outer arms and abdomen. Patients with cellulite and striae should be informed that liposuction will not improve these conditions. Other skin abnormalities, such as post-inflammatory dyschromia and keloidal or hypertrophic scarring, may become exacerbated by surgery. Abdominal scars should be assessed for fibrous bands, which may limit cannula maneuvering, and hernias, which put the patient at risk for abdominal viscus perforation. Physical structural components, such as musculoskeletal asymmetries, should also be noted and described to the patient as potential limitations to final contouring results.

All findings, particularly abnormal, should be thoroughly discussed with the patient, documented, and diagrammed in the medical record using a body diagram. Photographs or diagrams with outlines of treatment areas, as agreed upon with the patient and attested to by his or her signature, are useful to ensure the correct surgical sites on the day of the procedure. Preoperative and postoperative photographs taken at regular intervals—typically every three months for one year—are critical to confirm the outcome of the procedure, especially in patients with subtle results.

Typical volumes of aspirate—both adipose and fluid—and adipose tissue alone are approximately 1740 and 1160 cc, respectively (29). It is recommended

Table 4.10 Region-Specific Techniques

Location	Positioning	Infusion	Suctioning	Miscellaneous
Neck (chin, cheeks, jowls) (61–63)	Chin elevated/head extended (approximately 10° to 20°)	0.1% lidocaine tumescent solution using 1.5-inch, 25-gauge needle; avoid overinfusion to minimize compression of vital structures (particularly in the buccal region); allow 20–30 minutes prior to suctioning; entry points: submental at lateral mandible, lateral to jowls	Maintain shallow entry to avoid platysmal puncture (thin in older patients); danger zones: marginal mandibular nerve (care to avoid injury within 2 cm of mandibular border; elevate cannula away from underlying structures), spinal accessory nerve (lateral to anterior border of sternocleidomastoid); avoid oversuctioning of cheeks and jowl/cheek junction to reduce risk of dimpling)	Mark in seated upright position and note submental fat pad, jowls, mandibular border, anterior sternocleidomastoid, thyroid cartilage, and platysmal bands
Arms (65)	Lateral decubitus with arm lying over hips and rotated inward to expose posterior arm; lateral decubitus with forearm flexed, hand behind head, and elbow pointing away from face to expose posterior arm	0.1% lidocaine solution (if possible) using an infusion cannula; avoid excessive tumescence, which puts the patient at risk for compartment syndrome	Consider combining suctioning with anterior fat pad, but avoid the axillae because of many neurovascular structures; avoid oversuctioning but focus on creating a proportionate appearance	May have lax skin; do not oversuction, which can increase skin lining

(Continued)

Table 4.10 Region-Specific Techniques (*Continued*)

Location	Positioning	Infusion	Suctioning	Miscellaneous
Breast (female) (67,69,70)	Supine	0.1% lidocaine tumescent solution using an infusion cannula; entry points: two incisions in lateral axillary line and midinframammary crease	Lateral and inferior quadrants (suction in deep to midplane); upper quadrant (less removed because of flattening)	Typical candidate older than 45 years has fatty breasts; counsel on the possibility of some nipple elevation and loss of cleavage
Breast (male) (24,73)	Supine	0.1% lidocaine tumescent solution using 1.5-inch 25-gauge needle or infusion cannula; entry points at periphery of breast and inframammary crease; allow 20–30 minutes for vasoconstriction and diffusion prior to suctioning	Start with smaller cannulas (16-gauge Capistrano) for early tunneling, then a larger 14-gauge cannula; subareolar tissue may also be cautiously suctioned using shorter 16-gauge Capistrano cannulas	Be sure to evaluate for underlying causes of gynecomastia
Abdomen (66)	Supine, lateral decubitus (check for residual pockets)	0.1% lidocaine tumescent solution (periumbilical); entry points: 2–3 on lower and 2 on upper abdomen	Middle/deep fat layers (avoid superficial suction to prevent "draped" appearance or contour irregularities); use pinch/tent test to assess	Consider treatment of waist/hips to maintain relative proportions

Hips, outer thighs, buttocks (73)	Hips (lateral decubitus); outer thighs (lateral decubitus with wedge surgical pillow between legs; allows for anteriomedial rotation of femur similar to standing); buttock (prone)	0.05–0.075% lidocaine tumescent solution; entry points: approximately 4–5 placed equidistantly around the treatment area	Hip end point should be flat and not concave; care should be taken around the inferolateral gluteal crease (superficial suctioning to avoid damage to infragluteal ligaments; remaining buttock fat should be removed from middle to deep layers to avoid dimpling)	Critical to avoid oversuctioning (fat tunnels may not be completely emptied); focus should be on contour
Medial thighs and knees (65)	Lateral decubitus with superior thigh flexed cephalad overlying a brick-shaped pillow	0.1% lidocaine tumescent solution (upper medial thigh) and 0.05% for the remaining areas; entry points: approximately three—2 upper and 1 lower	Avoid circumferential thigh liposuction because of risk of lymphostasis if done in one procedure; avoid oversuctioning knee because of the risk of lymphatic injury and vascular damage	Mark area in a three-dimensional fashion to include the anterior, posterior, and medial thigh

that sessions be divided if anticipated combined aspirate (adipose and fluid) is greater than 4500 to 5000 cc or if multiple areas are to be treated. This is due to limitations on the amount of tumescent anesthesia that can be infused based on maximum lidocaine dose (35,36,38,41,74). When liposuction is divided into two or more sessions, treatment of adjacent regions—such as abdomen, hips/waist, and back or buttock, thighs, and knees—is recommended.

Surgical Unit

Outpatient tumescent liposuction is an extremely safe procedure when staff is well trained and appropriate equipment is utilized (Table 4.11). In comparison to the inpatient setting, outpatient liposuction is associated with a reduced rate of infection, decreased cost, and improved patient accessibility. To maintain safety of the procedure in the outpatient setting, the American Academy of Dermatology (AAD) liposuction task force has published a set of specific guidelines (Table 4.12) (74).

Tumescent Anesthesia

Preparation of tumescent anesthetic solutions should be completed on the day of the procedure by the surgical staff—preferably by the provider performing the liposuction—to reduce the possibility of errors (77,78–80).

Although it varies based on individual habitus characteristics, the amount of tumescent anesthetic may be estimated by treatment area (Table 4.13), while erring on the side of overestimating to make certain that enough anesthesia is available. The authors typically use a 0.05% tumescent solution for most areas, though a 0.1% tumescent solution is recommended for the upper inner thighs, periumbilical area, and for smaller liposuction procedures such as face and neck (78,80). Next, the total number of bags that may be used is calculated to ensure that the total lidocaine dosage is below the maximum dose (Table 4.14). Maximum doses may range from 35 to 55 mg of lidocaine per kilogram of body weight, with 35 mg/kg dosage recommended in patients taking medications that are metabolized by the cytochrome p450 system. In our practice, we recommend 45 mg/kg dosing for most patients and rarely use 55 mg/kg. Although the latter dosing is felt to be safe, we prefer to divide treatment into sessions to further improve the safety profile (8,12).

When preparing the tumescent solution, a methodical sequence is imperative to avoid errors. All saline bags are placed on one side; bags may be warmed prior to mixing using a microwave to reduce patient discomfort. The necessary components are drawn up sequentially and injected into a saline bag (Table 4.15). Bags are immediately labeled with the injected components and moved to the other side. Empty bottles or vials should be retained to verify that correct amounts have been mixed.

Table 4.11 Surgical Unit Recommendations

Surgical suite

- ○ Appropriate size (to accommodate personnel, patient, maneuverable surgical table, liposuction equipment, and allow access to all sides of the patient)
- ○ Surgical lighting
- ○ Scrub sink
- ○ Adjacent bathroom with shower and bench (postoperative cleansing and intraoperative patient use for urination because of the length of the procedure)

Operative equipment (76)

- ○ Comfortable, padded, maneuverable table (preferably electric/pneumatic)
- ○ Body positioning spacers
- ○ Sterile towels (for draping/fluid collection)
- ○ Warming pad or blanket (placed under the patient and covered with a sterile waterproof drape)
- ○ Emergency equipment
  - ▪ Advanced Cardiac Life Support cart including standard equipment such as a defibrillator, oxygen, continuous blood pressure monitor, and medications
  - ▪ Medications: 0.1 mg clonidine, 0.5–1.0 mg lorazepam, 25 mg fentanyl
- ○ Liposuction equipment
  - ▪ Aspiration pump (electric, closed circuit, overflow valve, disposable air filter, continuous suction) (75)
  - ▪ Infusion pump (electric, adjustable infusion speed)
  - ▪ Cannulas (* = recommended)
    - ● General
      - − Materials (stainless steel*, aluminum, deldrin, brass) (76)
      - − Structure (vary with respect to length, diameter, shape, and hole placement based on function)
      - − Size (<4.5 mm diameter, 2–3 mm diameter*) (74)
    - ● Infusion
      - − Cannula (small diameter, holes untapered)
      - − Needle (21- to 26-gauge, 1.5–2.5 in.) for smaller-volume procedures
    - ● Aspiration
      - − Aggressive (Becker, Capistrano, Cobra, Eliminator)
        - ● Tapered ends, distal holes
        - ● Greater risk of bleeding and soft tissue trauma
      - − Moderate (Fournier, Klein, Standard)
        - ● Blunted ends, proximal holes
        - ● Lower risk of bleeding and soft tissue trauma
  - ▪ Suction tubing
  - ▪ Tumescent solution components (also see Table 4.15)
    - ● 0.9% normal saline (500- and 1000-cc bags)
    - ● 2% lidocaine (50-cc vials)
    - ● 1:1000 epinephrine (1-cc vials)
    - ● 8.4% bicarbonate (25-cc vials)
    - ● 18-gauge needles
    - ● Syringes (1, 5, and 25 cc)

(Continued)

Table 4.11   Surgical Unit Recommendations (*Continued*)

o   IV setup
   ▪   IV pole and tubing
   ▪   18- to 21-gauge angiocatheter or butterfly kit
   ▪   Alcohol pads
   ▪   1 g Cefazolin (vial) or 300 mg Clindamycin (tablet)
   ▪   Sterile water (vial)
   ▪   0.9% normal saline (vial)
   ▪   Syringes (3 cc)
   ▪   OpSite dressings
   ▪   Surgical drape
o   Surgical scrub
o   Mayo stand
o   Surgical tray (suction/infusion cannulas, strabismus scissors, towels, towel clamp, sterile marking pen, sterile gauze, #11 blade, 5-cc syringe with 1% lidocaine with 1:100,000 epinephrine, 30-gauge ½-in. needle, gown)
Sterility
o   Technique (ensure all staff are trained, scrubbed, and clothed)
o   Clothing (surgical cap, masks, gloves, gown, and goggles)
o   Equipment (surgical tray, towels, blanket, drape, tubing)

Source: From Ref. 75.

Table 4.12   American Academy of Dermatology Liposuction Guidelines

Medical emergency algorithm
Training in management of cardiac emergencies (ACLS for liposuction surgeons and BLS for operating room staff)
Vital signs (pre- and postoperative): blood pressure and pulse rate
Capability of continuous cardiac, blood pressure, and pulse oximetry monitoring and availability of supplemental oxygen (procedures >100 cc of aspirate or with intravenous conscious sedation)

Table 4.13   Approximate Amounts of Required Tumescent Anesthesia

Neck/face: <250–500 cc
Abdomen: 1000–2500 cc
Back: 1000–2500 cc
Hips/waist: 1000–2000 cc
Buttocks: 1000–2000 cc
Outer thighs: 1000–2000 cc
Inner thighs: 1000–1500 cc
Lower outer buttocks: 1000–1500 cc
Knees: 250–500 cc

Table 4.14 Sample Calculation of Tumescent Anesthesia Volumes

A 70-kg patient is scheduled for liposuction on the outer/inner thighs, lower outer
    buttocks, and knees
Estimate of required solution: 3500 cc, 1500 cc, 500 cc (respectively), for a total of
    5500 cc
Maximum dose of lidocaine = 45 mg/kg × 70 kg = 3150 mg
1000-cc bag of 0.1% lidocaine = 1000 mg of lidocaine
1000-cc bag of 0.075% lidocaine = 750 mg of lidocaine
1000-cc bag of 0.05% lidocaine = 500 mg of lidocaine
Upper inner thighs require 500 cc of 0.1% solution = 500 mg
Remaining inner thigh/outer thigh require 3000 cc of 0.05% solution = 1500 mg
Lower outer buttocks require 1500 cc of 0.05% solution = 750 mg
Knees require 500 cc of 0.05% solution = 250 mg
Total required amount of lidocaine = 3000 mg
Alternatively, the maximum number of bags of 0.05% tumescent solution can be
    calculated by dividing maximum lidocaine dose by 500 mg
    (3150 mg/500 mg = 6.3 bags)

OPERATIVE SEQUENCE

The following timeline is a suggested sequence of steps that are required to
successfully and safely perform liposuction procedures.

Preoperative Period

Two to four weeks before surgery, the initial medical history should be reviewed
by the physician or a liposuction technician. Risks and potential adverse effects
specific to liposuction should be discussed at this time. These may include
infections, hematoma or seroma formation, nerve damage, skin necrosis, as well
as reactions to tumescent anesthesia including tachycardia, arrhythmias, and

Table 4.15 Tumescent Anesthesia Components

Lidocaine
    0.1% solution: 50 cc of 2% lidocaine per 1-liter bag
    0.075% solution: 37.5 of 2% lidocaine per 1-liter bag
    0.05% solution: 25 cc of 2% lidocaine per 1-liter bag
Epinephrine
    1:1,000,000–1:2,000,000
        The author of this chapter uses 0.65 mg of 1:1000 per 1-liter bag to reduce the risk of
            tachycardia
Bicarbonate
    1:10 ratio of bicarbonate to lidocaine
        5 cc of 8.4% bicarbonate for 0.1% 1-liter solution
        3.75 cc of 8.4% bicarbonate for 0.075% 1-liter solution
        2.5 cc of 8.4% bicarbonate for 0.05% 1-liter solution

possible death. Patients should be educated regarding medications, herbal supplements, and foods to avoid, if necessary. The appropriate blood work should be ordered at this time. Preoperative weight and measurements are obtained and treatment areas are documented and photographed. Finally, the surgical fee, partial or complete, is collected.

All blood work should be completed one week before surgery and reviewed by the treating physician. Any abnormal findings should be addressed.

The day before surgery, the physician performs the final review of medical history and calculates tumescent anesthesia requirements. The surgical suite is prepared for the procedure. The patient should be advised to consume a regular meal and to take 0.5 to 1.0 mg of lorazepam prior to sleep.

On the day of surgery, the patient should consume a regular breakfast and have a designated driver bring him or her to the office. An additional 0.5 to 1.0 mg of lorazepam should be taken 1 hour prior to procedure. Tumescent anesthesia should be prepared by the physician before patient arrival to the office.

Surgical Preparation

Upon arrival, the patient is greeted by the liposuction technician and checked in. A urine pregnancy test is administered and patient is asked to don a gown. Vital signs, including heart rate, respiration rate, pulse oximetry, and blood pressure, are obtained. If blood pressure is greater than 100/70 mmHg, 0.1 mg of clonidine may be administered by mouth, which assists with relaxation and prevents epinephrine-associated tachycardia. In addition, although baseline readings are always recommended, intraoperative monitoring with pulse oximetry and blood pressure may be needed if sedative medication is administered or in patients with cardiac or hypertensive history (74,81). An electrocardiogram is recommended to assess for abnormalities, such as undiagnosed ventricular ectopy, that may be exacerbated by epinephrine. If discovered, mild cases may be pretreated with a β-blocker, though severe cases may have to be canceled.

A physical examination is completed, including cardiac, pulmonary, and abdominal examination, as well as examination of the extremities. In higher-risk patients, such an examination should be completed prior to the day of surgery. Next, consent verification and "time-out" are used to confirm the correct patient, procedure, and surgical site, as required by the Joint Commission on Accreditation of Hospitals. A heating blanket is turned on and an intravenous (IV) line is started for medications and possible replacement fluids, if needed. One gram of cefazolin is then administered intravenously over 5 minutes, followed by a 3-cc IV flush.

At this point, the patient is ready to don sterile liposuction undergarments and a betadine surgical scrub is used on the treatment area and adjacent skin surfaces while the patient is standing. Likewise, the physician dons a surgical

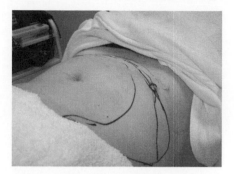

Figure 4.3 Treatment area marked with an indelible marker.

cap, mask, and goggles and begins personal surgical scrub, followed by a surgical gown and gloves. Treatment areas are then marked using a sterile surgical marking pen, confirming marked areas with the patient (Fig. 4.3). Also, infusion cannula entry sites are marked based on the ability to access all treatment areas using the least number of sites.

The patient is positioned on the procedure table and sterile towels and drape are applied around treatment sites. Sterile infusion tubing and an infusion cannula are attached to the infusion pump and tumescent solution is allowed to run through the tubing until air has been evacuated. Finally, sterile suction tubing is attached to the aspiration machine.

Tumescent Anesthesia Infusion

At this point, the infusion is ready to begin. Infusion cannula entry sites are anesthetized with 1% lidocaine with 1:100,000 epinephrine and small incisions are made using a #11 blade. Such incisions should be large enough for the cannula to pass without stretching the opening. An infusion cannula is placed in the subcutaneous adipose plane. For smaller volume liposuction cases of the face, neck, and knees, a 25-gauge, 1½-inch needle may be used instead. If difficulty with entry through the incision is encountered, strabismus scissors may be used to bluntly dilate the opening; if difficulty persists, entry into the subcutaneous space, as opposed to dermal tissue, should be verified. To this effect, the cannula is inserted vertically and only angled acutely once a "pop" or a release into the adipose tissue is noted. The cannula is advanced until infusion holes are covered by the skin. The infusion is then started at the rate of 25 to 125 cc/min (corresponding to 2 and 3 on a Klein pump) (80). This will result in an average infusion time of 1.5 to 2 hours for moderate volume removal. A liposuction assistant turns the machine on and off as requested and carefully records volumes infused into each area. Slower rates of infusion should be used in areas such as the face, neck, and arms to prevent excessive pressure on

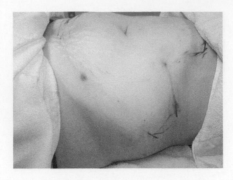

Figure 4.4 Treatment area infiltrated with anesthesia to approximately 1 cm outside of marked area.

vasculature, nerves, or airway. Infusion rate may also be limited by patient's pain tolerance (80), which may be mitigated by warming the tumescent solution or via distraction with music, dialogue, and vibration. However, if the patient is unable to tolerate the slowest infusion rate, conscious sedation with 25 mg of IV fentanyl with appropriate monitoring may be required.

The cannula is slowly advanced through the infused area as tumescence is noted, which manifests as induration and swelling with a slight *peau d'orange* and blanched appearance. Small "pops" of the infusion cannula may be noted as it is advanced through fibrous septae, sometimes requiring increased force or a change in angle. Infusion is performed in a fanning motion, beginning with the most lateral aspect of the treatment area and sequentially moving more medially. With each arm of the fan, infusions in a deep and superficial plane are required, sometimes necessitating two passes in the same location. Infusion should be extended 1 cm beyond marked area to ensure adequate anesthesia (Fig. 4.4). Alternate infusion entry sites may be required if the targeted treatment area is not completely infiltrated.

If tachycardia is encountered, it may be caused by either pain or epinephrine. Patient should be questioned regarding his or her level of pain and, if not significant, the tachycardia is likely related to the epinephrine. Some of the methods used in our practice to decrease the incidence of tachycardia due to epinephrine include using 0.65 mg instead of 1 mg of epinephrine per 1000 cc of tumescent solution and premedication with 0.1 mg of clonidine in patients with blood pressure greater than 100/70 mmHg, as noted previously.

Liposuction Procedure

Liposuction begins at the completion of the infusion process, starting with the area that was infused first. A minimum of 15 minutes should pass following the

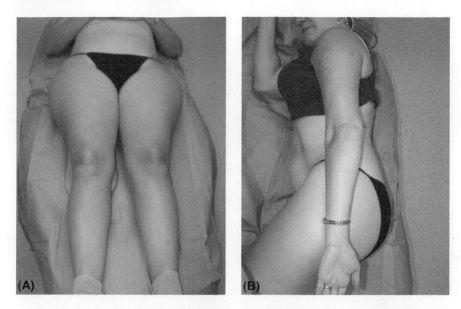

Figure 4.5 Abdomen: (**A**) supine and (**B**) lateral.

infusion process prior to suctioning to enhance aspirate quality. The patient is properly positioned to ensure optimal removal (Figs. 4.5–4.8). For the abdomen, the patient should be placed supine and lateral; for the arms, lateral and Klein-bent arm; for inner thigh by positioning pillow for high-step position and finishing with a frog-leg position; and for outer thigh by positioning pillow wedge between the thighs while in a lateral position. OpSite dressings

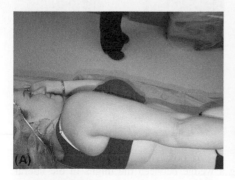
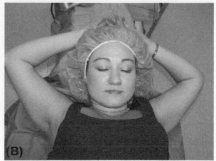

Figure 4.6 Arms: (**A**) lateral and (**B**) Klein-bent arm.

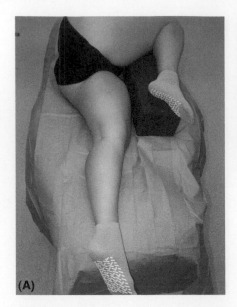
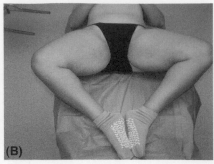

Figure 4.7 Inner thigh: (**A**) positioning pillow for high-step position and (**B**) finish frog-leg position.

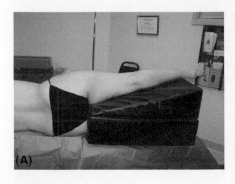
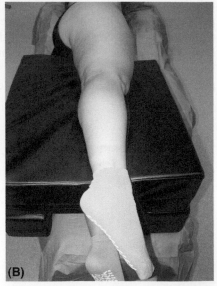

Figure 4.8 (**A, B**) Outer thigh: positioning a wedge between the thighs in the lateral position.

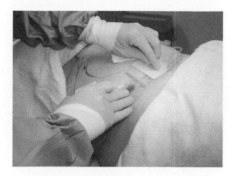

Figure 4.9 OpSite is placed over an infusion port.

(Smith & Nephew, London, U.K.) are placed over the infusion sites and a new stab incision is made (Fig. 4.9). This helps to prevent cutaneous trauma from repetitive cycling of the cannula through a port (Cox SE, personal communication).

For large adipose deposits, a thin, aggressive cannula (Capistrano) is used first to "break up the fat"; a larger cannula is then employed to debulk the adipose tissue; finally, the small cannula is reintroduced to aggressively thin the mid and upper planes. In fibrous areas, such as the back or the abdomen, an aggressive, small-diameter cannula (Capistrano) is utilized first and, as adhesions are relaxed and tunnels are created, a moderate cannula with a larger diameter (e.g., 3 mm) may then be used. In soft areas, such as those of the inner thigh or neck, less aggressive, smaller cannulas should be employed.

The cannula is inserted through a port when the aspirator is off, ensuring that the cannula label (flat surface of lock) faces up. This directs suction openings away from the dermis and toward the adipose layer. The port may need to be reopened with strabismus scissors in order for the cannula to pass. The aspirator is then turned on. Tunneling is performed in a deep plane using the active hand while the passive hand is overlying the skin, feeling the advancement of the instrument. The cannula is advanced completely and then retracted to the location of aspiration holes without exposure to the skin surface. The motion is repeated in a fanning or crisscross fashion to ensure even removal of fat. In soft areas or as the skin becomes progressively more pliable, an assistant may need to apply lateral traction with a flat hand to facilitate cannula movement. Alternate entry ports may be used as needed to maximize the removal of tissue, while less aggressive cannulas may be utilized as a pocket empties. The quality of fat should be monitored during aspiration. Yellow, low-fluid aspirate indicates a proper plane (Fig. 4.10); blood-tinged or frank-blood aspirate should prompt a switch of planes, ports, or cannula to a less aggressive one.

Persistent patient sensitivity during aspiration may be handled by switching to an alternate port or to a smaller-diameter cannula. Also, treatment

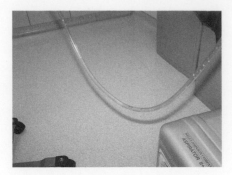

Figure 4.10 Proper lipoaspirate should be yellow in color with minimal blood-tinged fluid.

areas may be reinfused with 0.1% lidocaine solution—commonly used with inner thighs and periumbilical area—or even directly with 1% lidocaine. IV sedation with 25 mg of fentanyl under appropriate monitoring may also be used.

Completion of the procedure is indicated by the achievement of one or more surgical end points. These include aspiration of primarily blood-tinged fluid with minimal aspirate of fat, the pinch test, and the tent test. For the pinch test, skin is grasped between the thumb and the index finger to assess for a decrease in thickness (Fig. 4.2). During the tent test, the aspirator is turned off and the inserted cannula is lifted away from the body to assess the breadth of the surrounding skin. This should be even (Fig. 4.11); any irregular fat pockets should be touched-up as needed and the assessment should be repeated in a

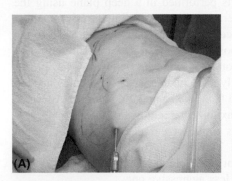
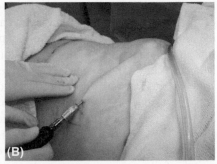

Figure 4.11 Tent test: (**A**) preprocedure and (**B**) postprocedure. Note the enhanced visibility of cannula following the removal of fat.

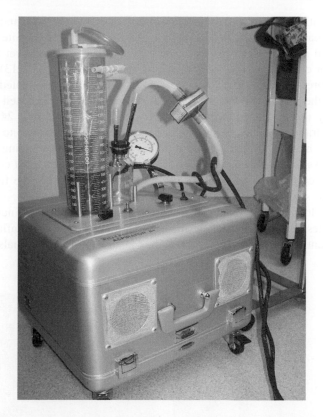

Figure 4.12 Lipoaspirate composed of adipose tissue (*top*) and fluid (*bottom*).

fanning motion throughout the treatment area. The volume of aspirate is recorded for each region before proceeding to the next area and sides are compared to ensure appropriate symmetry (Fig. 4.12).

IMMEDIATE POSTOPERATIVE CARE

Following the liposuction procedure, the patient gradually resumes an upright position. Initially, the head of the table is raised and the patient sits with his or her feet dangling for several minutes to minimize the risk of orthostatic hypotension. The IV fluid is left in place in case of a vasovagal reaction. In such an event, IV fluid in the form of normal saline is administered, the patient is placed in the Trendelenberg position, and vital signs are assessed. In severe cases or for prophylaxis in susceptible individuals, 0.3 mg of IV atropine can also be administered (82).

The patient is then lead to the shower and advised to cleanse and to gently compress treatment areas with a towel to express residual fluid. OpSite dressings are removed and absorbent pads or sanitary napkins are placed over the ports, with tape or elastic bandages used to secure them in place (Fig. 4.13).

Compressive garments appropriate for the region being treated are then donned by the patient (Fig. 4.14). Bimodal compression, as suggested by Klein, is generally recommended, with heavy compression for the first 24 hours to encourage drainage, followed by mild compression for the next two to four days (83). Others have advocated compression for longer durations ranging from one to four weeks, with an average of two weeks (77). In addition, cool compresses may be placed over the garment for 20 minutes every hour for the first day to reduce pain, swelling, bruising, and inflammation (84–90).

After drainage has stopped, petrolatum ointment is applied to incision sites and bandages are used to occlude the wounds until healed. Postinflammatory hyperpigmentation can develop at these sites in susceptible individuals and may

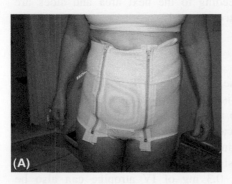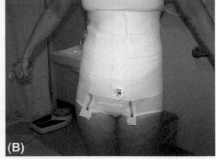

Figure 4.13 Port bandages: (**A**) sanitary napkin and (**B**) secured with tape.

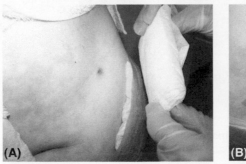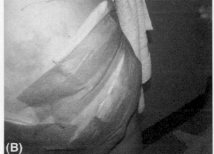

Figure 4.14 Compressive garments: (**A**) layer 1 and (**B**) layer 2.

take several months to resolve; 4% hydroquinone cream can be used to enhance clearing of such dyschromia.

Postoperative patient education is crucial to minimize patient worries and concerns and to ensure the best results with the lowest risk of adverse effects. A postoperative handout is given to and reviewed with the patient. Pain, typically described as soreness similar to that following an intense workout, should be minimal to moderate and may last several days. Fatigue for a few days is also common. Drainage is extensive for the first 24 hours and begins to slow over next few days. Contour irregularities may also be present initially, but usually resolve with decreased edema. Ecchymoses can be mild to extensive and are typically most prevalent around cannula sites. Dysesthesia is extremely common, but usually resolves over several months. Infection is rare, possibly because of the bacteriostatic properties of lidocaine (82,90). Nonetheless, if systemic symptoms and local signs of infection develop in the treatment area, oral or IV antimicrobial therapy with adequate coverage for methicillin-resistant staphylococcus may be necessary. Bacterial cultures should be obtained prior to initiating treatment. Hematomas and seromas are relatively uncommon, but may require drainage if they develop.

It is important that a postoperative call be placed the day after surgery to assess pain and drainage and to reassure the patient.

LONG-TERM POSTOPERATIVE CARE AND FOLLOW-UP

The first follow-up visit is usually scheduled for one week following liposuction. Subsequent follow-ups typically occur at 3, 6, and 12 months posttreatment. The patient should be advised that while a significant portion of the effects of the procedure will be noticeable within one week of treatment, the improvement will continue for up to one year as the skin retracts. Thus, touch-ups should not be performed within this period.

At each follow-up visit, photographs should be obtained for counseling and comparison. The patient should be reassured regarding retraction and fibrosis and educated on behavior modification, weight patterns, diet, and exercise.

Suboptimal outcomes may include limited improvement in appearance, asymmetry, and relative adiposity. Limited change after six to nine months is most common on the abdomen, possibly because of preoperative overestimation of fat in the subcutaneous versus visceral compartment or because of incomplete suctioning secondary to patient factors, such as poor pain tolerance or excessive blood in aspirate. Asymmetry may occur from discordant amounts of suctioning on each side or from unrelated musculoskeletal factors, such as scoliosis or muscle bulk (Fig. 4.15). Relative adiposity results from a relative increase in adipose deposits in a region adjacent to the treatment area, thereby causing a disproportionate contour. Ideally, this potential issue should be pointed out preoperatively, making the patient more accepting of additional procedures in the future.

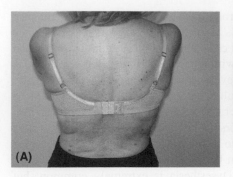 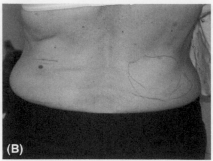

Figure 4.15 (**A**) Asymmetry due to scoliosis and (**B**) residual adiposity.

As noted previously, touch-ups should not be undertaken before the end of the one-year follow-up period. Although touch-up rates vary, one report in a busy liposuction practice noted an approximately 12% rate among both male and female patients, most commonly performed on the neck and the abdomen (91).

Prior to performing touch-ups, weight patterns should be assessed as a potential factor for the perceived suboptimal result. Reasonable goals need to be set for the touch-up procedure, as attempts to correct subclinical imperfections that the physician has difficulty detecting have a high probability of patient dissatisfaction. In all cases, the touch-up treatment should not be complimentary and the patient should be charged appropriate rates for the time and volume involved in the procedure.

CONCLUSIONS

With appropriate training, experience, and surgical setup, tumescent liposuction has proven to be a safe and effective treatment option for the management of unwanted fat. Careful patient selection, preoperative assessment, surgical technique, and postoperative care are paramount to the success of the procedure.

REFERENCES

1. Pitanguy I. Trochanteric lipodystrophy. Plast Reconstr Surg 1964; 34:280–283.
2. Schrudde J. Lipexheresis liposuction for body contouring. In: Grazer F, ed. Clinics Plastic Surgery. Vol 11. Philadelphia: WB Saunders, 1984:445–456.
3. Fischer G. Liposculpture: the "correct" history of liposuction, part I. J Dermatol Surg Oncol 1990; 16:1087–1089.
4. Fischer A, Fischer G. First surgical treatment for molding body's cellulite with three 5 mm incisions. Bull Int Acad Cosmet Surg 1976; 3:35.

5. Fournier P. Body Sculpturing Through Syringe Liposuction and Autologous Fat Re-injection. Paris: Samuel Rolf International, 1987.

6. Illouz Y. Body contouring by lipolysis; a 5 year experience with over 3000 cases. Plast Reconstr Surg 1983; 72:511–524.

7. Grazer F. Suction assisted lipectomy, suction lipectomy, lipolysis, lipexheresis. Plast Reconstr Surg 1983; 72:620–623.

8. Klein JA. Tumescent technique for regional anesthesia permits lidocaine doses of 35 to 55 mg/kg for liposuction: peak plasma are diminished and delayed 12 hours. J Dermatol Surg Oncol 1990; 16:248–263.

9. Klein JA. Tumescent technique for liposuction surgery. Am J Cosmet Surg 1987; 4:263–267.

10. Lillis PJ. Liposuction surgery under local anesthesia: limited blood loss and minimal lidocaine absorption. J Dermatol Surg Oncol 1988; 14:1145–1148.

11. Lillis PJ. The tumescent technique for liposuction surgery. Dermatol Clin 1990; 8:439–450.

12. Ostad A, Kageyama N, Moy RL. Tumescent anesthesia with a lidocaine dose of 55 mg/kg is safe for liposuction. Dermatol Surg 1996; 22:921–927.

13. Dolsky RL, Newman J, Fetzek JR, et al. Liposuction: history, techniques, and complications. Dermatol Clin 1987; 5:313–333.

14. Kesselring UK, Meyer R. Suction curette removal of excessive local deposits of subcutaneous fat. Plast Reconstr Surg 1978; 62:305–306.

15. Coleman WP III. The history of liposuction and fat transplantation in America. Dermatol Clin 1999; 17:723–727.

16. Alt TH, Coleman WP III, Skouge JW, et al. Guidelines of care for liposuction. Committee on Guidelines of Care. J Am Acad Dermatol 1991; 24:489–494.

17. Kloehn RA. Liposuction with "sonic sculpture": six years' experience with more than 600 patients. Aesthetic Surg Q 1996; 16:123–128.

18. Zocchi M. Ultrasound-assisted lipoplasty. Adv Plast Reconstr Surg 1998; 11: 197–221.

19. Lawrence N, Coleman WP III. Ultrasonic assisted liposuction: internal and external. Dermatol Clin 1999; 17:761–771.

20. Katz B, McBean J. The new laser liposuction for men. Dermatol Ther 2007; 2: 448–451.

21. The American Society for Dermatologic Surgery. Guiding principles for liposuction. Dermatol Surg 1997; 23:1127–1129.

22. Butterwick KJ, Goldman MP, Sriprachya-Anunt S. Lidocaine levels during the first two hours of infiltration of dilute anesthetic solution for tumescent liposuction: rapid versus slow delivery. Dermatol Surg 1999; 25:681–685.

23. Piveral K. Systemic lidocaine absorption during liposuction. Plast Reconstr Surg 1987; 80(4):643.

24. Klein J. The two standards of care for tumescent liposuction. Dermatol Surg 1997; 23:1194–1195.

25. Kucera IJ, Lambert TJ, Klein JA, et al. Liposuction: contemporary issues for the anesthesiologist. J Clin Anesth 2006; 18:379–387.

26. Bill TJ, Clayman MA, Morgan RF, et al. Lidocaine metabolism: pathophysiology, drug interactions, and surgical implications. Aesthet Surg J 2004; 24:307–311.

27. Tsai RY, Lai CH, Chan HL. Evaluation of blood loss during tumescent liposuction in Orientals. Dermatol Surg 1998; 24:1326–1329.

28. Bernstein G, Hanke CW. Safety of liposuction: a review of 9,478 cases performed by dermatologists. J Dermatol Surg Oncol 1988; 14:1112–1114.
29. Hanke CW, Bullock S, Bernstein G. Current status of tumescent liposuction in the United States: national survey results. Dermatol Surg 1996; 22:595–598.
30. Coleman WP III, Hanke CW, Lillis P, et al. Does the location of the surgery or the specialty of the physician affect malpractice claims in liposuction? Dermatol Surg 1999; 25:343–347.
31. Housman TS, Lawrence N, Mellen BG, et al. The safety of liposuction: results of a national survey. Dermatol Surg 2002; 28:971–978.
32. Coldiron B. Office surgical incidents: 19 months of Florida data. Dermatol Surg 2002; 28:710–713.
33. Coldiron B, Schreve E, Balkrishnan R. Patient injuries from surgical procedures performed in medical offices: three years of Florida data. Dermatol Surg 2004; 30:1435–1443.
34. Coldiron BM, Healy C, Bene NI. Office surgery incidents: what seven years of Florida data show us. Dermatol Surg 2007; 34:1–8.
35. Joint American Academy of Dermatology/American Society of Dermatologic Surgery Liaison Committee. Current issues in dermatologic office-based surgery. J Am Acad Dermatol 1999; 41:624–634.
36. Drake LA, Ceilley RI, Cornelison RL, et al. Guidelines of care for liposuction. Committee on Guidelines of Care. J Am Acad Dermatol 1991; 24:489–494.
37. Flynn TC, Narins RS. Preoperative evaluation of the liposuction patient. Dermatol Clin 1999; 17:729–734.
38. Butterwick J. Liposuction: consultation and preoperative considerations. In: Narins RS, ed. Safe Liposuction and Fat Transfer. New York: Marcel Dekker Inc., 2003: 41–67.
39. Kelley L. Lidotoxic at low lidocaine levels. Detroit, MI: World Congress on Liposuction, 2000.
40. Currier JS, Havlir DV. Complications of HIV disease and antiretroviral therapy. Int AIDS Society USA 2000; 2:16–20.
41. Klein JA. Thrombosis and embolism. In: Klein JA, ed. Tumescent Technique, Tumescent Anesthesia & Microcannular Liposuction. St Louis, MO: Mosby, 2000:67–78.
42. Eggleston ST, Lush LW. Understanding allergic reactions to local anesthetics. Ann Pharmacother 1996; 30(7–8):851–857.
43. Hernandez C, Emer J, Robinson JK. Perioperative management of medications for psoriasis and psoriatic arthritis: a review for the dermasurgeon. Dermatol Surg 2008; 34:446–459.
44. Chang LK, Whitaker DC. The impact of herbal medicines on dermatologic surgery. Dermatol Surg 2001; 27:759–763.
45. Butterwick KJ. Should dermatologic surgeons discontinue hormonal therapy prior to tumescent liposuction? Dermatol Surg 2002; 28:1184–1187.
46. Brown S, Cropfield O. The case for a lower dose pill: assessing the impact of estrogen dose. ORGYN 1995; 2:36–39.
47. Peverill RE. Hormone therapy and venous thromboembolism. Best Pract Res Clin Endocrinol Metab 2003; 17:149–164.
48. Lidegaard O, Edstrom B, Kreiner S. Oral contraceptives and venous thromboembolism: a five-year national case-control study. Contraception 2002; 65:187–196.

49. Drife J. Oral contraception and the risk of thromboembolism: what does it mean to clinicians and their patients? Drug Saf 2002; 25:893–902.
50. Spalding KL, Arner E, Westermark PO, et al. Dynamics of fat cell turnover in humans. Nature 2008; 453:783–787.
51. Brownell KD, Rodin J. Medical, metabolic, and psychological effects of weight cycling. Arch Intern Med 1994; 154:1325–1330.
52. Pasman WJ, Saris WH, Westerterp-Plantenga MS. Predictors of weight maintenance. Obes Res 1999; 7:43–50.
53. Skender ML, Goodrick GK, Del Junco DJ, et al. Comparison of two-year weight loss trends in behavioral treatments of obesity: diet, exercise, and combination interventions. J Am Diet Assoc 1996; 4:342–346.
54. Wing RR, Greeno CG. Behavioral and psychosocial aspects of obesity and its treatment. Baillieres Clin Endocrinol Metab 1994; 8:689–703.
55. McCargar LJ. Can diet and exercise really change metabolism? Medscap Womens Health 1996; 1:5.
56. Atkins RC. Dr. Atkins' New Diet Revolution. New York: HarperCollins, 2002.
57. Rabast U, Schönborn J, Kasper H. Dietetic treatment of obesity with low and high carbohydrate diets: comparative studies and clinical results. Int J Obes 1979; 3: 201–211.
58. Rabast U, Vornberger KH, Ehl M. Loss of weight, sodium and water in obese persons consuming a high or low carbohydrate diet. Ann Nutr Metab 1981; 25: 341–349.
59. McInnis KJ. Exercise and obesity. Coron Artery Dis 2000; 11:111–116.
60. Ozgur F, Tuncali D, Guler-Gursu K. Life satisfaction, self-esteem, and body image: a phychosocial evaluation of aesthetic and reconstructive surgery candidates. Aesthetic Plast Surg 1998; 22:412–419.
61. Kamer FM, Binder WJ. Avoiding depressions in submental lipectomy. Laryngoscope 1980; 90:1396–1400.
62. Jacob CI, Kaminer MS. Surgical approaches to the aging neck. In: Narins RS, ed. Safe Liposuction and Fat Transfer. New York: Marcel Dekker Inc., 2003:197–214.
63. Goddio AS. Suction lipectomy: the gold triangle at the neck. Aesthetic Plast Surg 1992; 16:27–32.
64. Kamer FM, Minoli JJ. Postoperative platysmal band deformity: a pitfall of submental liposuction. Arch Otolaryngol Head Neck Surg 1993; 119:193–196.
65. Klein JA. Anesthesia. In: Klein JA, ed. Tumescent Technique, Tumescent Anesthesia & Microcannular Liposuction. St Louis, MO: Mosby, 2000:174, 381, 297–324, 357–391, 427–439.
66. Narins RS. Abdomen, hourglass abdomen, flanks, and modified abdominoplasty. In: Narins RS, ed. Safe Liposuction and Fat Transfer. New York: Marcel Dekker Inc., 2003:95–119.
67. Gray LN. Liposuction breast reduction. Aesthetic Plast Surg 1998; 22:159–162.
68. Short K, Ringler SL, Bengtson BP, et al. Reduction mammoplasty: a safe and effective outpatient procedure. Aesthetic Plast Surg 1996; 20:513.
69. Matarasso A, Courtiss EH. Suction mammoplasty; the use of suction lipectomy to reduce large breasts. Plast Reconstr Surg 1991; 87.709–717.
70. Kaminer MS. Breast Liposuction in Liposuction Course. San Francisco: American Academy of Dermatology, 2003.

71. Samdal F, Kleppe G, Amland PR, et al. Surgical treatment of gynecomastia. Scand J Plast Reconstr Hand Surg 1994; 28:123–130.
72. Bermant M. Gynecomastia—dynamic technique. In: Narins RS, ed. Safe Liposuction and Fat Transfer. New York: Marcel Dekker Inc., 2003:215–234.
73. Cox SE. Violin: hips, outer thighs, and buttocks. In: Narins RS, ed. Safe Liposuction and Fat Transfer. New York: Marcel Dekker Inc., 2003:121–148.
74. Coleman WP, Glogau RG, Klein JA, et al. Guidelines of care for liposuction. J Am Acad Dermatol 2001; 45:438–447.
75. Monheit GD. The surgical suite for the liposuction surgeon. In: Narins RS, ed. Safe Liposuction and Fat Transfer. New York: Marcel Dekker Inc., 2003:19–28.
76. Bernstein G. Instrumentation for liposuction. Dermatol Clin 1999; 14:735–749.
77. Hanke W, Cox SE, Kuznets N, et al. Tumescent liposuction report performance measurement initiative: national survey results. Dermatol Surg 2004; 30:967–978.
78. Klein JA. Ancillary pharmacology. In: Klein JA, ed. Tumescent Technique. St Louis, MO: Mosby, 2000:196–209.
79. Jacob CI, Kaminer MS. Tumescent anesthesia. In: Narins RS, ed. Safe Liposuction and Fat Transfer. New York: Marcel Dekker Inc., 2003:29–40.
80. Narins RS, Coleman WP III. Minimizing pain for liposuction anesthesia. Dermatol Surg 1997; 23:1137–1140.
81. Klein JA, Kassarjdian N. Lidocaine toxicity with tumescent liposuction: a case report of probable drug interactions. Dermatol Surg 1997; 23:1169–1174.
82. Klein JA. Miscellaneous complications. In: Klein JA, ed. Tumescent Technique, Tumescent Anesthesia & Microcannular Liposuction. St Louis, MO: Mosby, 2000:43–60.
83. Klein JA. Postliposuction care: open drainage and bimodal compression. In: Klein JA, ed. Tumescent Technique, Tumescent Anesthesia & Microcannular Liposuction. St Louis, MO: Mosby, 2000:281–293.
84. Landry GL, Gomez JE. Management of soft tissue injuries. Adolesc Med 1991; 2:125–140.
85. Knight KL. Cryotherapy: Theory, Technique, and Physiology. Chattanooga: Chattanooga Corp, 1985.
86. Farry PJ, Prentice NG, Hunter AC, et al. Ice treatment of injured ligaments: an experimental model. N Z Med J 1980; 91:12–14.
87. El Hawary R, Stanish WD, Curwin SL. Rehabilitation of tendon injuries in sport. Sports Med 1997; 24:347–358.
88. Knight ATC. Cold as a modifier of sports-induced inflammation. In: Leadbetter WB, Buckwalter JA, Gordon SL, eds. Sports-Induced Inflammation: Clinical and Basic Science Concepts. Park Ridge: American Academy of Orthopaedic Surgeons, 1990:463–478.
89. Karunakara RG, Lephart SM, Pincivero DM. Changes in forearm blood flow during single and intermittent cold application. J Orthop Sports Phys Ther 1999; 29:177–180.
90. Klein JA. Antibacterial effects of tumescent lidocaine. Plast Reconstr Surg 1999; 104:1934–1936.
91. Lawrence L, Butterwick KJ. Immediate and long-term postoperative care and touch-ups. In: Narins RS, ed. Safe Liposuction and Fat Transfer. New York: Marcel Dekker Inc., 2003:329–341.

5

Lasers and similar devices

Bruce E. Katz and Jason C. McBean

INTRODUCTION

Unwanted fatty tissue is frequently associated with dissatisfaction in body shape and compromised self-esteem. Despite optimal dietary and exercise regimens, certain body areas such as the abdomen, flanks, thighs, back, and submental regions remain difficult to shape. Consequently, the public and medical demand for minimally invasive techniques that reduce excess adipose tissue continues to increase. Dermatologic surgeons remain at the forefront of research on newer and safer techniques that reduce downtime, complications, pain, and swelling.

Several new laser and light devices help reduce the risk and discomfort of surgery and patients often prefer these less invasive alternatives even at the possible risk of reduced efficacy. These include focused ultrasound, low-level laser therapy (LLLT), water jet–assisted liposuction (WAL), ultrasound-assisted lipoplasty (UAL), laser lipolysis, and cryolipolysis.

Noninvasive ultrasound that disrupts fat cells is popular among patients seeking to improve their shape by reducing adipose tissue in a safe and painless way without downtime. LLLT, a noninvasive method to reduce fatty tissue, was used a decade ago in conjunction with traditional liposuction to ease the removal of adipose tissue. It has experienced resurgence in recent years as a stand-alone, more gradual approach to fat reduction. WAL is a technique utilizing high infiltration pressure to separate tissue planes, which theoretically reduces trauma and volume of anesthetic fluid necessary to remove fatty tissue. UAL is a technique for removing fat by applying ultrasonic energy to emulsify adipose tissue. Laser lipolysis is another advance in the evolution of body contouring. During laser lipolysis, the laser directly interacts with adipose tissue, liquefying the fat and facilitating its removal. The laser energy also denatures collagen, creating a wound-healing cascade, whereby new collagen is created with subsequent skin tightening, particularly in areas with increased skin laxity.

Cryolipolysis is a noninvasive selective process whereby fat cells are reduced using localized, controlled cooling.

BACKGROUND

History of Medical Sonography and High-Intensity Focused Ultrasound

Sonography (ultrasound) is widely used in medical applications for diagnostic as well as therapeutic purposes. Diagnostic ultrasound is perhaps the most well-known function of medical ultrasound being used in many subspecialties. In obstetrics and gynecology, it is now a standard component of prenatal care, providing important information regarding fetal development during pregnancy. It is frequently used in cardiology to image chambers of the heart and surrounding vasculature. In gastroenterology, it may be used to visualize the spleen, liver, pancreas, and to diagnose appendicitis.

Therapeutically, ultrasound is being used to clean teeth and to generate regional heat and mechanical changes in physical and occupational therapy of the musculoskeletal system. Additionally, ultrasound has been used in urology to reduce kidney stones by lithotripsy and in ophthalmology to treat cataracts in a process called phacoemulsification. Focused ultrasound is also being used to generate localized heat to treat cysts, benign and malignant tumors, and, most recently, for the treatment of unwanted fat. This process is referred to as high-intensity focused ultrasound (HIFU), where frequencies lower than those used for diagnostic purposes are employed, yet significantly higher energies are administered to the tissue.

The term "ultrasound" refers to high-frequency acoustic energy beyond the audible range of human hearing. The audible range of sound is between 20 and 20,000 Hz. Beyond 20,000 Hz is a frequency higher than the human ear can detect. HIFU makes use of ultrasonic waves as carriers of energy propagated through human tissue. The basic premise of HIFU-induced tissue change is generation of hyperthermia. As ultrasonic waves are focused on a targeted region, acoustic pressure is rapidly elevated near a focus where tissue temperatures rise to a level that is sufficient for thermotherapeutic effects, subsequently resulting in coagulation necrosis (1).

The earliest use of the biological effects of HIFU was recognized in 1927, when Wood and Loomis observed changes such as searing of the skin, rupturing of red blood cells, and the lethal effects on mammals with a 200 to 500 kHz high-intensity ultrasound (2). In the 1930s, unfocused, low-intensity ultrasound was used for physiotherapy. In 1942, Lynn and colleagues showed that focusing ultrasound on a targeted region could produce highly localized effects (3). In the 1950s, focused ultrasound was used for brain therapy and subsequently attempted for the treatment of Parkinson disease (4). A resurgence in focused ultrasound occurred in 1994, when the first report of HIFU treatment for prostate cancer was published (5).

Low-Level Laser Therapy and Low-Level Laser Liposuction

In recent years, the use of LLLT has been advanced to treat a variety of conditions, including acute and chronic pain and injured tissues. In 2002, the U.S. Food and Drug Administration (FDA) approved low-level laser for the management of musculoskeletal pain. Additional studies have demonstrated LLLT's effect on cellular reactions. LLLT has been shown to (i) regenerate erythrocytes, enhancing their oxyphoric function; (ii) enhance fertilization potential of spermatozoa; (iii) stimulate the differentiation of stem cells; and (iv) improve wound healing (6–9).

In 2002, Neira et al. irradiated surgical sites with a 635-nm, 10-mW diode laser. Results demonstrated that 6 minutes after laser exposure, 99% of fat was released from adipocytes. Transmission electron microscopic images showed a transitory pore and complete deflation of the adipocytes (10). The surrounding nonadipocyte cells remained intact, demonstrating specificity for fat cells.

Neira et al. then studied the effects of LLLT via MRI evaluation of irradiated tissue to assess the depth of penetration within the subcutaneous layer (11). Results demonstrated less defined superficial adipose layer, less defined septae, and more coalescent adipose tissue. Jackson and colleagues applied LLLT externally prior to a liposuction procedure (12). The objective of Jackson's study was to determine whether LLLT impacted the procedure or patient recovery experience. The study noted that, for LLLT-treated patients, a greater volume of fat was extracted. In addition, patients experienced a reduction in postoperative edema and pain. Finally, when blinded physicians were asked to rate their ease of extraction, the emulsified fat induced by the laser treatment was found to be removed easily.

Water Jet–Assisted Liposuction

Power water–assisted liposuction is a variation of traditional liposuction that forces high-pressure fluid into the treatment area. The theory behind WAL is that the high-pressure fluid administered subcutaneously separates tissue planes more gently and assists in the removal of fatty tissue. During the procedure, a fan-shaped jet is directed at the subcutaneous space to separate adipose tissue. While the high-powered saline solution is being injected, it is simultaneously removed under defined vacuum pressure, along with the detached adipocytes. In contrast with traditional tumescent anesthesia, the fluid does not need to infiltrate for any particular length of time in order for the anesthetic or the epinephrine to take effect. As a result, a smaller volume of anesthetic fluid is required when administered with the power water–assisted device.

Ultrasound Assisted Lipoplasty

Ultrasonic systems have been used for more than 25 years for various medical and surgical procedures. In the 1980s and 1990s, Scuderi and Zocchi first used ultrasonic energy to emulsify and remove fat. One objective of using ultrasound technology was to increase tissue selectivity, making the aspiration more fat specific (13). By emulsifying the fatty tissue, the work of the surgeon was also diminished.

Three generations of UAL exist. The first-generation device (SMEI, Italy) emitted a frequency of 20 kHz. It delivered continuous ultrasound through solid, blunt-tipped probes 4 to 6 mm in diameter to pretreat fat before evacuation. Complications such as skin burns and dysesthesias from this early device led to the formation of a joint task force of the leading aesthetic and plastic surgery societies in 1995 to evaluate the merits, safety, and efficacy of UAL (14). Didactic and hands-on teaching courses were subsequently offered via the task force; however, complications remained.

Second-generation devices, Lysonix (Misonix, Farmingdale, New York, U.S.) and Contour Genesis (Mentor, Santa Barbara, California, U.S.), used frequencies of 22.5 and 27.0 kHz, respectively. Both devices utilized hollow cannulas that would simultaneously emulsify and aspirate adipose tissue; however, probe tips were thick, requiring large incisions of up to 1 cm in length, with a lumen of only 2 mm. The small lumen size made aspiration slow and, in turn, increased the duration that the ultrasonic energy interacted with adipose tissue. These shortcomings contributed to postprocedural seromas and burns.

In 2001, a third-generation ultrasonic system, known as the vibration amplification of sound energy at resonance (VASER), was introduced by Sound Surgical Technologies (Louisville, Colorado, U.S.). The VASER improves on many of the shortcomings of the first- and second-generation devices. This system operates at a frequency of 37.5 kHz, thereby increasing the efficiency of ultrasound delivery. In addition, a new concept of pulsed delivery of ultrasonic energy was introduced with this device. Pulsed ultrasound reduces the energy delivered to tissue by up to 50% compared with previous UAL systems. Additionally, the newly designed probes are grooved to redistribute the energy, transferring some of the vibration energy from the front of the tip to a region proximal to the tip. A variety of tube sizes allow for flexibility when treating fibrous versus nonfibrous areas and large versus smaller areas, including areas previously unsuitable for traditional UAL such as the arms, submental region, and thighs. There is still controversy about this technology due to the need for large incisions to accommodate the probes, risk of burns, and lack of evidence for skin tightening.

Laser Lipolysis

Laser lipolysis is an aesthetic procedure that employs a laser fiber, which interfaces directly with subcutaneous adipose tissue, leading to its emulsification. Based on both selective thermolipolysis and controlled thermodenaturation of collagen (with water serving as tissue chromophore), the following findings have been documented: (*i*) liquefaction of fatty tissue, (*ii*) coagulation of blood vessels, (*iii*) induction of collagenesis, and (*iv*) promotion of tissue tightening by clinical evaluation after thermal injury (Figs. 5.1 and 5.2) (15).

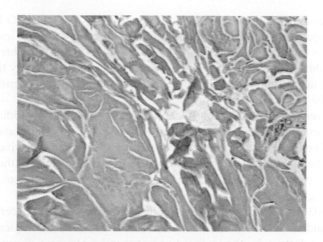

Figure 5.1 Photomicrograph following laser lipolysis. Note the thickened collagen bundles. (H&E), original magnification 100x.

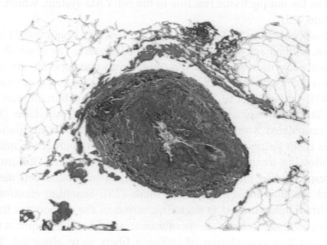

Figure 5.2 Photomicrograph following laser lipolysis. Note the obliteration of a small arteriole in subcutis. (H&E), original magnification 100x.

Dressel performed the first laser lipolysis procedure in 1990 on a 34-year-old man with unwanted abdominal adiposity (16). Apfelberg then published the first description of the direct action of laser in fatty tissue, that is, laser lipolysis, in 1992 (17). In 1994, Apfelberg et al. conducted the first multicenter trial that studied laser-assisted liposuction. The device was a 40-W Nd:YAG laser used with a 0.2-second pulse duration and equipped with a 600-μm fiber inserted into a 4- or 6-mm cannula. Cold saline was used for cooling. The laser fiber was fully encased within a cannula and was not in direct contact with the fatty tissue. The study suggested a trend toward decreased ecchymoses, pain, and edema, and less strain for the physician (18).

Between 2000 and 2003, Blugerman, Schavelzon, and Goldman introduced the concept of pulsed 1064-nm Nd:YAG laser in laser-assisted liposuction. Their work serves as the foundation of the current principles and techniques behind laser lipolysis by being the first to demonstrate the effect of laser energy on fat, as well as the surrounding dermis, vasculature, and apocrine and eccrine glands (19–22).

In 2003, Badin supported these findings in a study titled "Laser lipolysis: flaccidity under control." The author demonstrated several histological changes after thermal damage by the laser: adipocyte membranes were disrupted, blood vessels were coagulated, and new collagen was reorganized. These histological changes translated to the clinical observation of decreased local adiposities, reduced ecchymoses and blood loss, and improved skin tightening. Badin concluded that laser-assisted lipolysis was less traumatic because of smaller cannula size as well as the unique tissue reaction to the Nd:YAG system, which improved skin retraction (23).

A subsequent study by Goldman et al. treated 1734 patients, 313 men and 1421 women, with an age range between 15 and 78 years. The study showed less blood loss and ecchymoses, improved patient comfort postoperatively, and better efficacy for reducing fat in denser areas, such as those seen in gynecomastia (24).

In 2005, Ichikawa et al. evaluated freshly excised human skin and subcutaneous fat, which was irradiated with a pulsed Nd:YAG laser. A control group was cannulated with only the hand piece without laser irradiation. Hematoxylin and eosin staining as well as scanning electron micrograph images were obtained following treatments. Histological findings included 300-μm tunnels, which corresponded to the laser fiber diameter, disintegrated cell membranes, small vessel coagulation, and dispersed lipids (25). Scanning electron microscopy after irradiation showed greater destruction of the adipocytes than in the control group. Degenerated cell membranes, vaporization, liquefaction, carbonization, and heat coagulation of collagen fibers were observed. The study concluded that laser-assisted lipolysis appeared to be histologically effective for the destruction of human fat tissue.

In a 2006 study, Kim and Geronemus used magnetic resonance imaging (MRI) to evaluate the volume of fat reduction after laser lipolysis. In addition to the 17% fat volume reduction documented by MRI, patients noted a 37% improvement in only three months, quick recovery times, and good skin retraction (26).

In October 2006, the U.S. FDA approved a 1064-nm Nd:YAG laser (SmartLipo, Cynosure, Westford, Massachusetts, U.S.) for the surgical incision,

Table 5.1 Laser Lipolysis Devices

Device Name	Manufacturer	Lasing Medium	Wavelength (nm)
SmartLipo	Cynosure	Nd:YAG	1064
CoolLipo	CoolTouch	Nd:YAG	1320
ProLipo	Sciton	Nd:YAG	1064/1319
LipoLite	Syneron	Nd:YAG	1064
Lipotherme	Osyris	Diode	980
SlimLipo	Palomar	Diode	924/975
SmoothLipo	Eleme	Diode	920
SmartLipo MPX	Cynosure	Nd:YAG	1064/1320

excision, vaporization, ablation, and coagulation of soft tissues (27). In 2008, Katz and McBean published the first study reviewing potential complications in 537 consecutive laser lipolysis cases using a 1064-nm Nd:YAG system. There were no systemic adverse events and only five local complications, which included four skin burns and one local infection, resulting in a complication rate of less than 1%. They also identified a 3.4% touch-up rate, which is well below the 12% previously reported in liposuction literature. At the time of publication, more than 50 articles on laser lipolysis were identified via PubMed literature search and 9 new laser lipolysis devices have been introduced and aggressively marketed (Table 5.1). As the technology continues to advance, improved efficacy is sure to follow.

Cryolipolysis

Cryolipolysis is a technology in its infancy that extrapolates the well-known sequelae of cold exposure on fatty tissue—panniculitis. The brief history involves a 2008 preliminary porcine study by Manstein and colleagues. Using a cold copper applicator, chilled by an antifreeze solution at $-7°C$ for 5 to 21 minutes, Manstein et al. demonstrated lobular panniculitis and several-millimeter loss of subcutaneous fat, which occurred gradually over 3.5 months. Histological findings at 30 days demonstrated smaller and variously sized adipocytes, as well as abundant lipid-laden macrophages engaging in phagocytic activity. Gross vertically cut tissue from Yucatan pig tissue showed approximately 40% fat reduction at 3.5 months following cold exposure treatment (28).

The cooling device, known as Zeltiq (Zeltiq Aesthetic Inc., Pleasanton, California, U.S.), is FDA approved for noninvasive fat reduction. Preliminary human studies have demonstrated a reduction in the superficial fat layer thickness, ranging from 20% to 80% following a skin cryolipolysis treatment (29). Although limited in the amount of fat reduction achievable, the technology has become quite popular.

CURRENT STATE OF KNOWLEDGE

Focused Ultrasound

Objective of Treatment

The goal of HIFU is to effectively treat unwanted fatty tissue in the most minimally invasive manner. Liposuction is one of the top four most common cosmetic surgical procedures performed today and it is still regarded as the criterion standard for fat removal with respect to efficacy. However, for some patients, the prospects of liposuction are either too daunting physically or economically or are medically contraindicated. As long as patient expectations are kept low, HIFU is an excellent alternative for those patients who are not liposuction candidates.

HIFU is an alternative for patients who desire body contouring without the risk of liposuction because the procedure is performed without penetrating the skin barrier. There are two HIFU systems currently used for the removal of fatty tissue: UltraShape (UltraShape, Yoqneam, Israel) and Liposonix (Medicis, Scottsdale, Arizona, U.S.). UltraShape was the first ultrasonic device to show noninvasive selective fat cell destruction (30). With the UltraShape device, energy is administered at a controlled depth using a nonthermal pulsed wave. The mechanical acoustic effects of UltraShape cause selective fat cell disruption without injury to skin vessels, nerves, or connective tissue (31,32).

Liposonix contrasts with UltraShape in that it has an adjustable depth of penetration and produces heat. The Liposonix device delivers both high-intensity and high-frequency ultrasound energy to target subcutaneous fat. It achieves targeted reduction of adipose tissue by thermocoagulation of adipocytes. A transducer delivers energy across the skin surface at low intensity and delivers a high-intensity, sharp focus in the subcutaneous fat.

Both devices rely on the body's natural inflammatory response, whereby macrophages are recruited to the treatment area to engulf and transport lipids and cell debris away. The breakdown products are then transported through the blood, gradually absorbed, and delivered via the lymphatic system to the liver, where they are processed through physiologic metabolic pathways. No change in free fatty acids, total cholesterol, very low-density lipoprotein, high-density lipoprotein, low-density lipoprotein, or triglyceride levels has been reported.

At print, neither device is approved for use in the United States; however, if the FDA approves these devices, they may experience a significant market success by filling a void within the body sculpting industry for an effective noninvasive technology that reduces unwanted fatty tissue.

Indications and Patient Selection

As in all aesthetic procedures, a history and physical examination is an integral component of treating our patients. Patients with a history of any implantable devices, including a pacemaker, defibrillator, cardiac stent, or abdominal surgery such as hernia repair using a mesh, are strictly contraindicated. In addition, history of abdominal wall hernia, previous abdominal surgeries, or cardiac conditions such as uncontrolled hypertension, ischemic heart disease, and congestive heart failure, also contraindicate HIFU procedures. Patients with liver disease, infectious hepatitis, HIV, coagulopathy, or excessive bleeding are not ideal candidates. Clearly, pregnant or lactating women should be excluded from treatment. Patients should not be taking medications that interrupt the coagulation cascade, such as aspirin, nonsteroidal anti-inflammatory drugs, clopidogrel, and warfarin.

Physical examination will be important in determining the degree of expected improvement. Managing patient expectations is particularly crucial with HIFU treatments because the results may be subtle. Many clinicians use commercially available pinch calipers containing a measurement scale for baseline adiposity measurement as well as for estimating the number of treatments. Patients with fat deposits between 2 and 5 cm should be considered for treatment, while those with fat deposits of 6 cm or more should be excluded because of little to no improvement. Areas with adiposities less than 2 cm are not suitable for HIFU treatments. Body mass index (BMI) should also be less than 35 kg/m^2 and patients should be within 10% of their ideal body weight. Some practices complete a body composition analysis, which measures weight, BMI, and body fat percentage, prior to treatment. The clinician should also assess for abdominal or thoracic surgical scars, as the elevated enthusiasm or motivation for patients to undergo these procedures may cause them to omit important information from their historics.

Treatment Algorithm—UltraShape

Prior to treatment, informed consent is obtained and the patient is photographed. Waist circumference and tissue thickness should be measured and recorded. The patient is marked in the upright position to properly identify treatment areas under the effect of gravity. It is important to verify that the marked area is greater than 2.0 cm. The patient is positioned supine with arms at his or her sides. Drapes are then placed on the periphery of the marked areas to better delineate and isolate treatment location.

Cooled castor oil, which serves as a coupling medium, is applied to the skin before and during treatments. The cooled oil also enhances patient comfort and can be readministered throughout the procedure. Treatment parameters are preset and a transducer delivers a focused ultrasonic beam at a mean frequency of 200 ± 30 kHz with an acoustic output intensity of 17.5 W/cm^2. These preset parameters ensure selective damage to fat cells within the treatment area.

An intelligent video tracking and guidance system ensures that the treatment is performed only on the designated treatment area, that the entire area is covered homogenously, and that every point is treated only once. The operator will continually move the transducer until the tracking system indicates "end of treatment."

Optimizing Outcomes

As mentioned previously, it is imperative that patient expectations are managed and that excellent preoperative photographs and measurements are obtained to compare and contrast them to the posttreatment results. In addition to photographic documentation, circumference measurements, fat thickness measurements by caliper, and subject satisfaction questionnaires have been used to document efficacy. The expected reduction in thickness by caliper measurement is 3 to 6 mm per treatment session (33). The average waist circumference reduction may range between 2 and 3.95 cm (34). Sessions can be spaced between one and four weeks.

With regard to safety and adverse events of the device, mild erythema is expected. There have been reports of postinflammatory hyperpigmentation, neurosensory loss, blisters, bruising, edema, and pain, along with lack of results. Laboratory assessments, such as CBC, lipid profile, BUN/Cr, and thyroid and liver function tests, have been performed in studies and demonstrate no significant changes. HIFU treatment for fat removal is yet to be approved by the FDA and further studies are required to clarify the cause of and to assist in reducing the incidence of adverse events and to improve efficacy.

Low-Level Laser Therapy

Although an increasing number of studies evaluated the effects of LLLT through the early 2000s, controversy remains regarding the efficacy of this treatment at a clinical level. In 2009, Jackson and colleagues again set out to evaluate the effects of LLLT for fat reduction. In their latest study, they evaluated the efficacy of LLLT as a stand-alone noninvasive procedure for body contouring. In a double-blind, randomized, placebo-controlled trial, 67 subjects underwent treatments with either the LLLT device or a sham treatment three times per week for two weeks. Circumference measurements were obtained from treatment areas, which included the waist, hip, and bilateral thighs, at baseline and on completion of the treatments. Patients in the treatment group showed a statistically significant reduction of 3.51 in. in total circumference across all three sites compared with control subjects who revealed a 0.684-in. reduction. Jackson and colleagues concluded that LLLT can reduce the overall circumference measurements of treated regions (35). At present, there are no other studies that evaluate the safety and efficacy of LLLT for body contouring.

Recently, a device named Zerona (Erchonia, Santa Barbara, California, U.S.) became commercially available. At the time of publication, Zerona does not have the FDA 510(k) market clearance; however, information is available via their Web site and the device has been featured on popular television programs and other media outlets as "the first noninvasive body contouring procedure to effectively remove excess fat." To our knowledge, no studies have documented clinical efficacy of the Zerona device and Jackson's study is the only double-blind, placebo-controlled evaluation of a similar device utilizing LLLT technology.

Water Jet–Assisted Liposuction

There is little literature evaluating the safety and efficacy of the power water–assisted method available in peer-reviewed journals. In 2007, a European study by Araco evaluated postoperative pain of power WAL versus traditional liposuction (36). Sixty patients were enrolled in their study. Thirty-two patients were treated with power WAL (Body-Jet, Human Med, Schwerin, Germany) and 28 patients were treated with traditional tumescent liposuction. Postoperative pain was assessed by two methods. The first was a visual analogue scale (VAS), where patients were asked to rank the pain on a scale from 0 (no pain) to 10 (maximum pain). The second method involved counting the number of analgesic pills consumed daily by the patient, as recorded in the medical chart. The development of ecchymoses was also evaluated by two independent plastic surgeons.

After four days, 87% of patients treated with the WAL device were pain free versus 3.6% of patients who were treated with traditional liposuction. Ecchymoses were less prominent in patients who underwent power WAL. Although an interesting concept, it is difficult to extrapolate strong evidence from this one study for the typical liposuction candidate. There is concern regarding the tolerability of this procedure under local anesthesia because of the minimal anesthetic incubation time during the simultaneous infiltration and suctioning.

Another study by Stutz and Krahl evaluated the effects of WAL for patients with lipoedema (37). The aim of the study was to determine the effects of WAL on lymph vessels, blood vessels, and adipocytes in patients suffering from lipoedema of the lower extremities. They concluded that, although it is traditionally risky to treat lipoedema patients with liposuction because of possible damage to lymphatic tissue, the WAL technique was gentle enough to preserve this fragile vasculature. The aspirates from the 30 treated patients contained intact adipocytes (70%), intact small capillaries and venules, and no intact lymph vessels, suggesting selective safety for lymphatic vasculature when performed along the safe longitudinal axis of lymphatic flow. Through a series of immunohistochemical staining, the authors suggested that the three-dimensional expansion of the subcutaneous space that occurs with WAL allows the aspiration of adipose tissues with reduced shearing force, thus minimizing injury to blood and lymphatic vessels.

We are still missing adequate data and studies evaluating the safety and efficacy of the WAL procedure. The studies mentioned earlier are the only two identified with a PubMed literature search for water, jet, or high pressure assisted liposuction. These two studies evaluate specific attributes of the procedure; however, both lack depth with respect to patient selection, preoperative setup, operative technique, histological evaluation, postoperative management, long-term follow-up, and safety. Clearly, more studies are necessary in order for this procedure to truly become an accepted option for aesthetic surgeons and patients.

Ultrasound-Assisted Liposuction

Objective of Treatment

As mentioned in "Background" section of this chapter, UAL has significantly progressed since the first-generation devices. The latest VASER has minimized the risk of complications from earlier devices by using small-diameter probes with grooved tips and pulsed delivery of ultrasonic energy. The objective of treatment by the VASER device is the removal of unwanted fatty tissue while making the procedure safer and more effective for patients, as well as more predictable and less fatiguing for the surgeon.

Technical Considerations

The VASER platform is composed of an amplifier, which emits the ultrasonic energy, grooved probes and hand pieces, vented cannulas, aspirator, infiltration pump, and wireless foot switch for fluid infiltration and ultrasound activation. The platform is designed as a contiguous unit on wheels for improved mobility, ease of use, and compact surgical setup.

In contrast with previous ultrasonic devices, the grooved probe design redistributes the ultrasound energy, transferring some of the vibration energy from the front of the tip to a region just proximal to the tip. This design increases the efficiency of fragmentation or emulsification by allowing for smaller diameter probes. Probe sizes are selected based on treatment location. For example, large-diameter 3.7-mm probes are intended for larger treatment areas, while smaller probes (2.9 mm) should be considered for smaller volume areas. The number of grooves is also chosen based on treatment area, with one groove used for more fibrous tissue and three grooves used for the least fibrous fatty tissue.

Indications and Patient Selection

The VASER system is indicated for use in all primary lipoplasty procedures and is particularly helpful for treating fibrotic or dense areas, such as the back and hips. In addition to aesthetic lipoplasty, the procedure has been applied for the treatment of Madelung disease, Cushingoid-related buffalo-hump deformities, HIV-associated lipodystrophy, gynecomastia, and minimal-scar breast reductions (38).

The ideal candidates are those with no significant past medical histories, with realistic expectations, and with good skin tone with moderately sized local adiposities on physical examination. Patients who have had dramatic weight fluctuations or those who report poor nutritional status are not ideal candidates for the procedure. Candidates with loose skin, striae, or dramatic weight loss as seen following gastric bypass are better served with abdominoplasty procedures.

Treatment Algorithm

Once the ideal patient is selected and informed consent is obtained, photographs should be obtained. Preoperative photographs are imperative to demonstrate the results of the procedure and for medicolegal purposes. They also serve as excellent learning tools for the surgeon. Some surgeons post the preoperative photos in the operating room for comparison during surgery, since anatomic units may become distorted with tumescent anesthesia and with the loss of the effects of gravity in the supine position.

The patient is then marked in the anatomic, upright position, which also assists the surgeon in identifying surgical units throughout the procedure. Pre-existing scars and anatomical deformities should be identified for the patient so as to avoid potential confusion for complication from the surgical procedure. Incision sites are then marked. These sites should be placed in locations that are obscure, yet allow adequate access for the ultrasonic probes. For example, many surgeons place sites at the inferior and superior umbilical rims for access to inferior and superior abdominal regions, respectively. Strategic sites in areas typically covered by undergarments are also useful. Ideal locations allow for cross tunneling, which leads to even and consistent fatty tissue reduction.

Special skin protectors or skin ports are placed within the incision sites to shield the entrance sites from friction and possible heat generated by the vibratory and back-and-forth motion of the ultrasonic probe. Once tumescent anesthesia has been administered and the skin protectors have been placed, ultrasonic probes are then used to emulsify fatty tissue. Recommended energy settings are influenced by tissue type and are obtained from the manufacturer. Following administration of ultrasonic energy, aspiration is performed. The ease of adipose tissue removal is notable and may result in less fatigue and quicker aspiration of similar volumes when compared with traditional liposuction.

Surgical End Points

The end point of ultrasonic energy for fat emulsification is determined by feel and clinical judgment. When pinching the skin for fat thickness, it should feel more pliable than following tumescent anesthesia infiltration. The probe should easily glide through the subcutaneous tissue contrasting with the initial firmness. The skin should not become hot or warmer than the surgeon's hand. The surgeon may consider using an infrared thermometer to monitor skin surface temperatures. Some surgeons recommend that ultrasonic energy not be administered for longer than one minute per 100 mL of tumescent anesthesia; however, there is no substitute for clinical judgment and the surgeon should exercise caution instead of relying on manufacturer guidelines for end points.

Optimizing Outcomes

As with any tumescent liposuction procedure, uniform and complete tumescent fluid administration is important. During UAL, it is particularly important to infuse sufficient wetting solution to avoid rapid heating of the tissue, which may translate to thermal burns. Additionally, the probe should not be left in one location for too long to avoid direct contact with the dermis.

Side Effects and Complications

First- and second-generation devices suffered a tarnished reputation because of several reports of untoward side effects, including seromas, delayed resolution of swelling, painful dysesthesias, thermal burns, hyperpigmentation, and severe abdominal wall necrosis. The third-generation VASER device has demonstrated fewer complications (39). In a series of 77 patients, Jewell et al. identified excellent clinical outcome with no major complications after VASER-assisted lipoplasty. Jewell et al. noted that the aspirate contained 80% or greater supernatant fat, minimal blood loss, and infrequent edema or ecchymosis (40).

Latest Developments and Future Considerations

Newer indications for the VASER technology include treatment of hyperhidrosis, bromhidrosis, and high-definition liposculpture. Commons and Lim treated 13 patients with significant axillary hyperhidrosis or bromhidrosis with VASER ultrasound (41). Eleven of the 13 patients had significant reduction in sweat and odor and had no recurrence of significant symptoms at six months. No significant complications were noted. Postoperative pain was minimal, lasting one to two days, and a full return to basic activities occurred the day after the procedure.

VASER-assisted high-definition liposculpture was pioneered by Hoyos and Millard (42). The objective is to create a "chiseled appearance" by highlighting the three-dimensional muscular anatomy. The authors treated 306 patients with VASER ultrasound in a continuous mode for deep debulking and pulsed mode for the immediate subdermal plane. Superficial emulsification was performed to define the relevant anatomy for the muscle groups in each treatment area and additional fat over the muscles was removed. The authors found that VASER-assisted high-definition lipoplasty produced satisfactory results in 84% of patients. There were no reports of skin necrosis; however, there were 9 cases of port-site burns, 5 cases of prolonged swelling, and 20 cases of seromas, which is a rate higher than that seen with traditional high-definition liposculpture. These complications are likely due to the superficial nature of the VASER treatments.

Laser Lipolysis

Objective of Treatment

"Albert Einstein discovered that a tiny amount of mass is equal to a huge amount of energy; which explains why, as Einstein himself so eloquently put it in a famous 1939 speech to the Physics Department at Princeton, 'You have to exercise for a week to work off the thigh fat from a single Snickers'."

—*Dave Barry, Miami Herald Columnist*

The objective of treatment is, of course, the removal of unwanted fat—a continuous issue that has led many scientists in America to warn of an obesity epidemic. The demand for minimally invasive procedures that reduce fatty tissue continues to increase. Laser lipolysis is the latest advance in this effort. The primary indication for laser lipolysis is body contouring through the liquefication of localized deposits, as well as skin tightening via neocollagenesis. It is not, however, indicated for the treatment of obesity.

The advantages of laser lipolysis, when compared with traditional liposuction alone, have been detailed in many articles. To summarize, laser lipolysis liquefies adipose tissue, thus facilitating removal with smaller-sized cannulas (Fig. 5.3). In turn, this advantage may ease patient recovery by reducing postoperative pain, swelling, and bruising. The photothermal effect of the laser has also been shown to coagulate blood vessels, which may further reduce the risk of ecchymoses. These advances improve patient tolerance of the procedure and hasten return to daily activities (43).

The improvement of skin laxity was a controversial topic throughout the early stages of laser lipolysis development. To date, two studies have successfully corroborated the clinical observations suggesting skin tightening. DiBernardo et al. evaluated skin tightening after laser-assisted liposuction by measuring with a skin elasticity device, tattoo skin marking, and a three-dimensional camera (44). The average skin tightening index, or elasticity, increase was 26% and the average reduction in surface area, or skin shrinkage, was 17%. McBean and Katz

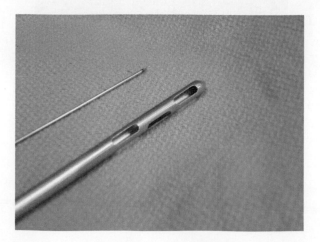

Figure 5.3 Laser fiber adjacent to traditional aspiration cannula.

used 4 × 4 cm temporary India Ink square tattoos to evaluate the skin tightening effects of a 1064/1320-nm device (45). An average of 18% reduction in the surface area of the squares was observed from baseline (Figs. 5.4 and 5.5).

Drawbacks linked to laser lipolysis include increased operator time, undercorrection due to inadequate cumulative energies, and the significant learning curve when first using the device. Results may, therefore, vary, with some studies indicating no difference when compared with traditional liposuction and others demonstrating superior results. As the technology and experience with these devices continue to evolve, the burden of these disadvantages may lighten. For example, newer-generation devices have cannulas allowing for simultaneous lasing and suctioning, thus reducing the original two-step nature of laser lipolysis and reducing operator time.

Indications and Patient Selection

The ideal candidate for laser lipolysis is a patient who is thin, in good health, and presents with isolated pockets of removable fat. Careful assessment and patient education is crucial prior to proceeding with the procedure. Candidates with too much fat are more likely not to experience dramatic results. All patients should be advised that laser lipolysis is not a substitute for healthy diet and exercise.

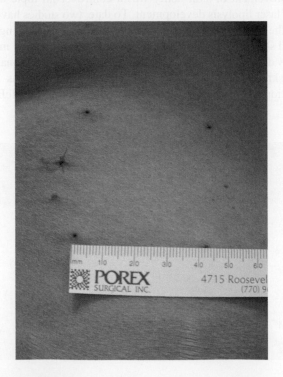

Figure 5.4   India Ink square tattoos before SmartLipo.

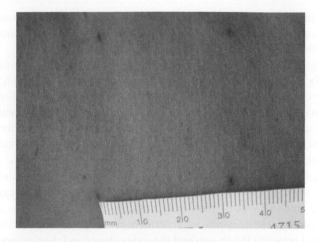

Figure 5.5 India Ink square tattoos after SmartLipo.

Laser lipolysis is indicated for any location that demonstrates unwanted fatty tissue and modest skin laxity. These include the submental area, upper arms, abdomen, back, hips, inner thighs, outer thighs, knees, calves, and ankles. Patients with irregularities or uneven areas after a previous liposuction or other surgical procedures such as abdominoplasties are excellent candidates.

During the patient interview, a full history should be obtained. Also, patient goals should be clearly identified. For instance, a patient may have a specific reason for undergoing laser lipolysis: "I have had this area since puberty and it has always bothered me"; "I diet and I exercise regularly; however, I cannot seem to lose this last area"; "I am getting married next weekend." The first two patients will have realistic expectations regarding their results, while the third will require education on the estimated timeline of treatment results. By evaluating the patient's motivation, the surgeon may better comprehend the likelihood of satisfaction from the procedure.

A good overall health is required for the procedure. Some practices obtain medical clearance for patients older than 60 years or for those with cardiovascular disorders, hypertension, or diabetes. Additionally, patients with liver disease, previous chemotherapy, and those on antiretroviral medications are at risk of impaired lidocaine metabolism and, subsequently, lidocaine toxicity. Medication allergies should be assessed. Patients should be provided with a list of medications to be avoided prior to the procedure. These include blood-thinning agents such as warfarin, clopidogrel, aspirin, and nonsteroidal anti-inflammatory drugs. Also, medications that inhibit cytochrome P450 liver enzymes, such as selective serotonin reuptake inhibitors and azole antifungal agents, can decrease lidocaine metabolism. Laboratory evaluation should include a hepatitis panel, complete blood count with differential, coagulation studies, HIV antibodies, pregnancy test, and serum electrolytes.

During physical examination, the patient should stand in a well-lit room wearing only a disposable paper bikini. In addition to the treatment area, the surrounding cosmetic units should also be assessed. For example, for optimum body contouring a patient may benefit from treatment of both abdomen and hips, while their initial concern may have only been their abdomen. Any irregularities, dimples, or scars should be pointed out and documented using photographs prior to the procedure, so they are not mistaken for postoperative defects.

It is essential to evaluate the quality of the skin tone. Although laser lipolysis can improve the skin tone, particularly where skin laxity is exaggerated, it may not be able to create a completely smoothened appearance. To assess skin tone and elasticity, the surgeon may perform a "snap test," where the skin is gently pinched between the thumb and the index finger and then released. Instant recoil indicates good skin elasticity, whereas slow recoil indicates poor elasticity. Other indications of poor skin quality include the presence of cellulite, dimples, fine wrinkling, and actinic damage. Nonetheless, one advantage of laser lipolysis is that improvement of skin tone is possible, whereas in traditional liposuction, these skin characteristics may sway the surgeon away from such candidates (Figs. 5.6–5.8).

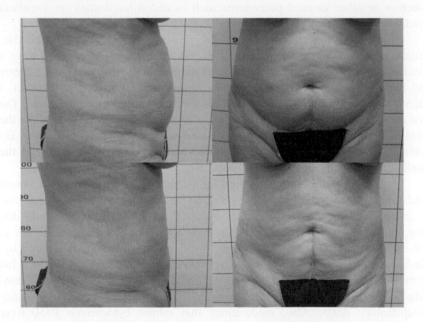

Figure 5.6 Laser lipolysis, before and after treatment of the abdomen.

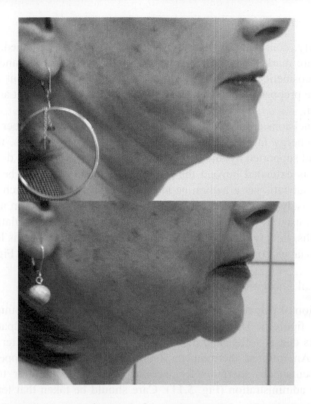

Figure 5.7 Laser lipolysis, before and after treatment of the submental area.

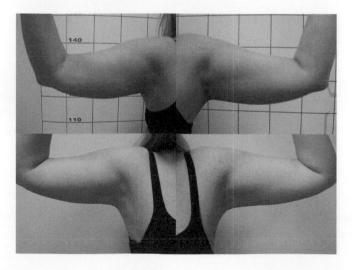

Figure 5.8 Laser lipolysis, before and after treatment of the arms.

Technical Considerations

Preoperatively, consent forms are signed, photographs are obtained, and treatment areas are marked. Treatment areas are marked to delineate landmarks and liposuction cosmetic units which become distorted with tumescent anesthesia. The areas are prepped with an antimicrobial cleanser and tumescent anesthesia is administered.

Tiny incisions are made in the skin and a 600-μm optical fiber is inserted to transmit energy into the subcutaneous tissue. In most devices, the fiber is carried in and supported by microcannulas of variable lengths. The distal portion of the fiber is extended beyond the end of the cannula and can be visualized through the subcutis via a helium-neon (He-Ne) laser source, which guides the surgeon precisely through the treatment areas (Fig. 5.9). A 1.5-mm adit or #11-blade stab is used to introduce the cannula, which is then manipulated through various depths, liquefying the adipose tissue. Once the fatty tissue is liquefied, it is removed via suction aspiration using 1.4- to 3.0-mm cannulas (Fig. 5.10).

Surgical End Points and Laser Energy

A combination of palpation and skin temperature are end points commonly used during laser lipolysis. During lasing, the tissue is continually palpated until it becomes less dense, softer, and more pliable than immediately after tumescent anesthesia. An infrared thermometer (some devices come equipped with an internal subcutaneous thermometer) should be used to monitor temperature during laser administration (Fig. 5.11). Care should be taken that temperatures

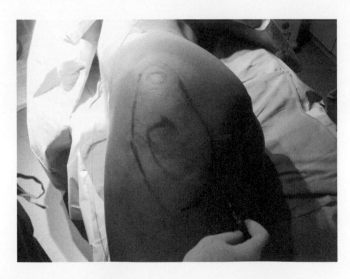

Figure 5.9 He:Ne beam, as visualized under the skin.

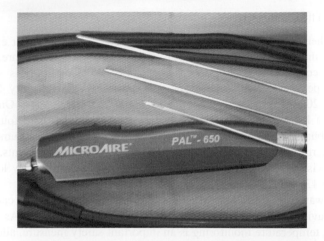

Figure 5.10 Aspiration cannulas.

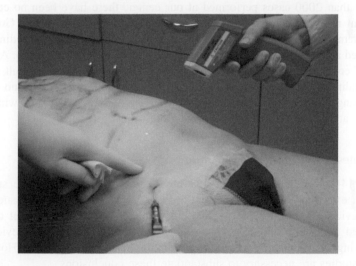

Figure 5.11 Infrared thermometer.

do not to exceed 38°C to 40°C. These temperatures are associated with improved skin contraction, wound healing, and retraction of skin to underlying tissue. However, as excessive heat is accumulated, the risk of tissue trauma and thermal injury is increased. Surface temperatures exceeding 47°C may result in epidermal and dermal injury (44). In our experience, keeping the skin surface temperature between 38°C and 40°C creates skin tightening while minimizing epidermal and dermal burns. Finally, additional end points, such as the accumulated energy, may be employed.

Side Effects and Complications

Although there are potential complications of laser lipolysis, in our experience with more than 2000 cases, the actual side effects have been rare. A 2008 report on complications associated with laser-assisted lipolysis evaluated 537 cases performed with tumescent anesthesia between January 2006 and November 2007 (45). There were no systemic adverse events. One patient developed a localized infection treated with oral antibiotics and four patients developed burns. The burns likely occurred secondary to a rapid accumulation of thermal energy localized to one area. Finally, out of 537 patients, only 19 required revisions—a touch-up rate of 3.5%, which is significantly lower than the 12% to 13% reported in previous liposuction literature.

One way to prevent thermal injury is to continually move the cannula and to avoid leaving the laser in one location for excessive durations. As discussed previously, temperature monitoring is an important safety measure, allowing the surgeon to maintain a range between 38°C and 40°C.

An additional safety concern is the theoretical possibility of nerve damage. In more than 2000 cases performed at our center, there have been no cases of persistent neuropathy, paresthesias, or numbness. Earlier studies by Goldman et al. demonstrated histologically intact nerve fibers with surrounding disintegrated adipose tissue, suggesting a selective thermolytic effect (46). Another issue of concern is the possibility of increased serum lipids as a result of lipolyzed adipose tissue. To this effect, Goldman and colleagues found no significant change in triglycerides and lipid profiles among patients treated with laser lipolysis at one day, one week, and one month postprocedure.

Latest Development and Future Considerations

A new 1444-nm device was recently approved by the FDA for the surgical incision, excision, vaporization, ablation, and coagulation of soft tissue. This latest device comes after the publication of a 2009 study by Tark et al. that suggested superior lipolytic effect of this wavelength over other devices by quantifying oil production and through histological evaluation (47). However, further studies are necessary to substantiate these conclusions.

Surgeons are now combining various procedures, such as fractional laser or radiofrequency devices, with laser lipolysis to create a synergistic effect of skin tightening. An additional laser lipolysis device (Smartlipo TriPlex Workstation, Cynosure, Westford, Massachusetts, U.S.) (Fig. 5.12) has been introduced to the market and uses three wavelengths: 1064, 1320, and 1440 nm. The objective behind incorporating three wavelengths in one system is to enhance the efficacy and rate of lipolysis and to improve skin tightening while reducing operative time. Safety measures, including a subcutaneous temperature-monitoring system and motion-sensing devices, have also been implemented to minimize overtreatment and thermal complications.

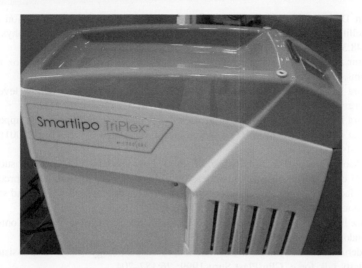

Figure 5.12 TriPlex workstation by Cynosure.

CONCLUSIONS

In the foreseeable future, additional laser and light devices will continue to advance in an effort to optimize patient safety and clinical efficacy. Current devices are already being investigated for additional purposes such as cellulite treatment, hyperhidrosis, facial sculpting, and periorbital adipose tissue and skin tightening. Future considerations will include more precise laser and light devices, improved technology, and a reduced side effect profile.

REFERENCES

1. Kim YS, Rhim H, Choi MH, et al. High intensity focused ultrasound therapy: an overview for radiologists. Korean J Radiol 2008; 9(4):291–302.
2. Wood RW, Loomis AL. The physical and biological effects on high frequency sound waves with great intensity. Philos Mag 1927; 14:417–436.
3. Lynn JG, Zwermer RL, Chick AJ, et al. A new method for the generation and use of focused ultrasound in experimental biology. J Gen Physiol 1942; 26:179–193.
4. Fry WJ, Fry FJ. Fundamental neurological research and human neurosurgery using intense ultrasound. IRE Trans Med Electron 1960; ME-7:166–181.
5. Madersbacher S, Pedevilla M, Vingers L, et al. Effect of high-intensity focused ultrasound on human prostate cancer in vivo. Cancer Res 1995; 55:3346–3351.
6. Siposan DG, Lukacs A. Relative variation of the received dose of some erythrocyte and leukocyte indices of human blood as a result of low-level laser irradiation: an in vitro study. J Clin Laser Med Surg 2001; 19:89–103.
7. Cohen N, Lubart R, Rubinstein S, et al. Light irradiation of mouse spermatozoa stimulation of in vitro fertilization and calcium signals. Photochem Photobiol 1998; 68:407–413.

8. Ben Dov N, Schefer G, Irintchev A, et al. Low-energy laser irradiation affects satellite cell proliferation and differentiation in vitro. Biochem Biophys 1999; 1448:372–380.
9. Tafur J, Mills PJ. Low-intensity light therapy: exploring the role of redox mechanisms. Photomed Laser Surg 2008; 26(4):323–328.
10. Neira R, Arroyave J, Ramirez H, et al. Fat liquefaction: effect of low level laser energy on adipose tissue. Plast Reconstr Surg 2002; 110(3):912–922.
11. Neira R, Jackson R, Dedo D, et al. Low-level laser-assisted lipoplasty: appearance of fat demonstrated by MRI on abdominal tissue. Am J Cosmet Surg 2001; 18(3): 133–140.
12. Jackson R, Roche G, Butterwick KJ, et al. Low-level laser-assisted liposuction: a 2004 clinical trial of its effectiveness for enhancing ease of liposuction procedures and facilitating the recovery process for patients undergoing thigh, hip and stomach contouring. Am J Cosmet Surg 2004; 21(4):191–198.
13. Katz B, Sadick NS, eds. Procedures in Cosmetic Dermatology: Body Contouring. London: Saunders Elsevier, 2009:123.
14. Fredericks S. Analysis and introduction of a technology: ultrasound-assisted lipoplasty talk force. Clin Plast Surg 1999; 26:187–204.
15. Sasaki G, Tevez A. Laser assisted liposuction for facial and body contouring and tissue tightening: a 2 year experience with 75 consecutive patients. Semin Cutan Med Surg 2009; 28:226–235.
16. Dressel T. Laser lipoplasty: a preliminary report. Lipoplast Soc Newsl 1990; 7:17.
17. Apfelberg D. Laser-assisted liposuction may benefit surgeons and subjects. Clin Laser Mon 1992; 10:259.
18. Apfelberg DB, Rosenthal S, Hunstad JP, et al. Progress report on multicenter study of laser-assisted liposuction. Aesthetic Plast Surg 1994; 18(3):259–264.
19. Blugerman G. Laser lipolysis for the treatment of localized adiposity and "cellulite." Abstracts of World Congress on Liposuction Surgery. Dearborn, Michigan, 2000.
20. Schavelzon D, Blugerman G, Goldman A, et al. Laser lipolysis. Abstracts of the 10th International Symposium on Cosmetic Laser Surgery. Las Vegas, Nevada, 2001.
21. Goldman A, Schavelzon D, Blugerman G. Laser lipolysis: liposuction using Nd: YAG laser. Rev Soc Bras Cir Plast 2002; 17:17–26.
22. Goldman A, Schavelzon D, Blugerman G. Liposuction using neodimium:yttrium-aluminum-garnet laser. Abstr Plast Recontr Surg 2003; 111:2497.
23. Badin AZ, Moraes LM, Gondek L, et al. Laser lipolysis: flaccidity under control. Aesthetic Plast Surg 2002; 26(5):335–339.
24. Goldman A, Shavelzon ED, Blugerman GS. Laser lipolysis: liposuction with Nd: YAG Laser. Rev Soc Bras Laser 2003; 2:335.
25. Ichikawa K, Miyasaka M, Tanaka R, et al. Histologic evaluation of the pulsed Nd: YAG laser for laser lipolysis. Lasers Surg Med 2005; 36:43–46.
26. Kim KH, Geronemus RG. Laser lipolysis using a novel 1,064 nm Nd:YAG Laser. Dermatol Surg 2006; 32(2):241–248.
27. U.S. Food and Drug Administration Web page. Available at: http://www.fda.gov/consumer/updates/liposuction082007.html. Accessed May 30, 2011.
28. Manstein D, Laubach H, Watanabe K, et al. Selective cryolysis: a novel method of non-invasive fat removal. Lasers Surg Med 2009; 40:595–604.
29. Nelson A, Wasserman D, Avram M. Cryolipolysis for reduction of excess adipose tissue. Semin Cutan Med Surg 2009; 28:244–249.

30. Coleman KM, Coleman WP, Benchetrit A. Non-invasive, external ultrasonic lipolysis. Semin Cutan Med Surg 2009; 28:263–267.
31. Brown SA, Greenbuam L, Shutmaster S, et al. Characterization of nonthermal focused ultrasound for noninvasive selective fat cell disruption (lysis): technical and preclinical assessment. Plast Reconstr Surg 1997; 23:1213–1218.
32. Moreno-Moraga J, Valero-Altes T, Riquelme M, et al. Body contouring by noninvasive transdermal focused ultrasound. Lasers Surg Med 2007; 39:315–323.
33. Katz B, Sadick NS, eds. Procedures in Cosmetic Dermatology: Body Contouring. London: Saunders Elsevier, 2009:116.
34. Teitelbaum SA, Burns JL, Kubota J, et al. Noninvasive body contouring by focused ultrasound: safety and efficacy on the Contour I device in a multicenter, controlled, clinical study. Plast Reconstr Surg 2007; 120:779–789.
35. Jackson R, Dedo D, Roche G, et al. Low-level laser therapy as a non-invasive approach for body contouring: a randomized, controlled study. Lasers Surg Med 2009; 41:799–809.
36. Araco A, Gravante G, Araco F, et al. Comparison of power water-assisted and traditional liposuction: a prospective randomized trial of postoperative pain. Aesthetic Plast Surg 2007; 31:259–265.
37. Stutz J, Krahl D. Water jet-assisted liposuction for patients with lipoedema: histologic and immunologic analysis of the aspirates of 30 lipoedema patients. Aesthetic Plast Surg 2009; 33:153–162.
38. Katz B, Sadick NS, eds. Procedures in Cosmetic Dermatology: Body Contouring. London: Saunders Elsevier, 2009:125.
39. Roustaei N, Lari S, Chalian M, et al. Safety of ultrasound-assisted liposuction: a survey of 660 operations. Aesthetic Plast Surg 2009; 33:213–218.
40. Jewell M, Fodor PB, de Souza Pinto EB, et al. Clinical application of VASER-assisted lipoplasty: a pilot clinical study. Aesthet Surg J 2002; 22:131–146.
41. Commons GW, Lim AF. Treatment of axillary hyperhidrosis/bromidrosis using VASER ultrasound. Aesthetic Plast Surg 2009; 33(3):312–323.
42. Hoyos AE, Millard JA. VASER-assisted high-definition liposculpture. Aesthet Surg J 2007; 27(6):594–604.
43. Goldman A, Gotkin RH. Laser-assisted liposuction. Clin Plast Surg 2009; 36: 241–253.
44. DiBernardo BE, Reyes J, Chen B. Evaluation of tissue thermal effects from 1064/ 1320 nm laser-assisted lipolysis and its clinical implications. J Cosmet Laser Ther 2009; 11(2):62–69.
45. McBean JC, Katz BE. A Pilot study of the efficacy of a 1064 and 1320 nm sequentially firing Nd:YAG laser device for lipolysis and skin tightening. Laser Surg Med 2009; 41(10):779–784.
46. Goldman A, Shavelzon D, Blugerman G. Laser lipolysis: liposuction using and Nd: YAG laser. Rev Soc Bras Cir Plast 2002; 17(1):17–26.
47. Tark KC, Jung JE, Song SY. Superior lipolytic effect of the 1444 nm Nd:YAG laser: comparison with the 1064 nm Nd:YAG laser. Laser Surg Med 2009; 41(10): 721–727.

6

Mesotherapy and injection lipolysis

Adam M. Rotunda

INTRODUCTION

Technological advances and established clinical techniques described in this book, as well as those currently under investigation, will each in some way redefine our approach to understanding and treating body fat. At one end of the body-shaping spectrum (Fig. 6.1) are conventional surgical procedures like abdominoplasty and liposuction, which have historically been the centerpiece to dramatic body contouring and which will likely remain the criterion standard for many years to come. On other end of the spectrum are novel light and energy sources (1) as well as injectable methods aimed at reducing and perfecting the curves on our bodies.

Injection lipolysis describes the subcutaneous placement of pharmacologically active, physiologically compatible detergents, such as bile salts, to chemically ablate fat. Injectable lipolytic techniques have been described as mesotherapy, but injection lipolysis differs from mesotherapy historically and with regard to the ingredients and injection techniques utilized (2).

Just as filler substances have satisfied a significant aesthetic need for restoring volume, an injectable product may have an analogous role in reducing unwanted tissue. There has been significant controversy in the medical and lay press about "injectable lipolysis," or Lipodissolve®, and "mesotherapy." Moreover, it is imperative to highlight that at the time of this writing, the use of the medications described in this chapter as a means to reduce fat is not approved by any regulatory authority. The ingredients discussed are primarily available from compounding pharmacies only, although this may change in the next several years pending approval in the European Union or by the Food and Drug Administration (FDA) in the United States of a pharmaceutical-grade medication indicated for "fat dissolution." Physicians are advised to inquire about the status of this procedure with their malpractice carrier, and become informed (and

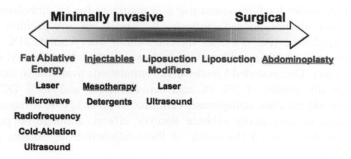

Figure 6.1 A spectrum of conventional surgical and innovative nonsurgical, minimally invasive procedures for reducing and contouring fat.

likewise appropriately consent patients) of the risks, benefits, and alternatives to this technique. In time, the core principles and mechanism of this novel technology may secure it as a proven technology that adds to our toolbox for the nonsurgical treatment of modest collections of subcutaneous fat.

BACKGROUND

Injectable fat treatments emerged internationally after Patricia Rittes, a dermatologist in São Paolo, Brazil, reported clinically significant reductions in infraorbital fat injected with Lipostabil® (3). Numerous investigators subsequently replicated the concept of localized fat reduction after injections of phosphatidylcholine (PC) and deoxycholate (DC) (the two principle ingredients in Lipostabil) in the upper thighs, abdomen, neck, dorsocervical region ("buffalo hump"), as well as lipomas (4–18). More recent, rigorous, double-blinded clinical trials have substantiated findings from the small, uncontrolled, open-label case series that prevailed in the earlier literature on the subject.

The recent popularity of injection lipolysis—and *la raison d'être* of this chapter in the book—can be attributed in part to direct-to-consumer marketing by commercial treatment centers, such as MedSculpt, and the branding of the injectable treatments as Lipodissolve. The relative notoriety of this procedure arises from the publicity surrounding untoward complications, national and international medical society warnings against the practice of this unregulated procedure, as well as state legislation that has banned or threatens to ban the procedure (19–25).

Lipodissolve and the medication typically used in injection lipolysis are not currently manufactured as an approved pharmaceutical agent, rather they are formulated and distributed by compounding pharmacies only. The standard ingredients are typically based on the original Lipostabil formulation. Lipostabil is manufactured by Sanofi-Aventis (Paris, France) and is approved in select

European countries for intravenous use as a treatment for fat embolism, dyslipidemia, and alcohol-induced cirrhosis. It consists of soy lecithin–derived phosphatidylcholine (PC, 5%), its solvent sodium deoxycholate (DC, 2.5%), dl-alpha-tocopherol (vitamin E), sodium hydroxide, ethanol, and benzyl alcohol, in sterile water. Compounded Lipodissolve formulations available in the United States typically consist of 5% PC and between 4.2% and 4.7% DC. Some pharmacies add caffeine, collagenase, carnitine, or other agents if requested by the physician to purportedly enhance lipolytic effects, although no published clinical data has verified the utility of these adjunctive ingredients for that purpose (26).

In contrast to injection lipolysis, *mesotherapy* describes an injection technique first introduced in 1952 by French physician Michel Pistor (2). Mesotherapy has been used in Europe for decades, primarily as a treatment for musculoskeletal pain and inflammatory conditions, as well as cellulite, photoaging, and scarring, among other conditions. The treatments typically consist of numerous epidermal, dermal, or subcutaneous injections of vasodilators, anti-inflammatory medications, herbs, hormones, antibiotics, enzymes, or coenzymes. Similar to injection lipolysis, this technique is not regulated, no pharmaceutical-grade formulations exist, and there are no standardized ingredients. Compounding pharmacies may offer premixed "cocktails" or individual injectable ingredients, which can be combined immediately before injection.

There is only limited published data demonstrating that mesotherapy (as defined traditionally in the previous paragraph) is effective for fat loss. Caruso and colleagues (27) have reported in vitro evidence that adipocytes incubated with isoproterenol, aminophylline, and yohimbe undergo lipolysis. Isoproterenol or another β_2-receptor agonist, which is purposely used to initiate an intracellular cascade leading to hormone-sensitive lipase activation, can theoretically induce fat cell reduction, *not* ablation. There is some evidence that isoproterenol may indeed be effective at reducing subcutaneous fat (28), but these data have not been replicated in studies with more than several patients. Additional clinical data are forthcoming.

In contrast to a belief of some practitioners, use of most ingredients in injection lipolysis and mesotherapy for fat loss is *not* considered "off-label." According to a statement released by the FDA about Lipodissolve:

> These are unapproved drugs for unapproved uses. . . . In virtually all cases, FDA regards compounded drugs as unapproved drugs, meaning — compounded drugs are not FDA-approved drugs. The use of compounded drugs is not considered "off-label" use. If a physician uses an FDA-approved drug for an indication not in the approved labeling this is considered "off-label" use. FDA approval of a drug includes approved labeling for use, and means that the FDA has evaluated the safety and efficacy of a drug for a specific use and population. Once approved, a drug may be prescribed by a licensed physician for a use that, based on the physician's

professional opinion, is appropriate. This prescribing is considered part of the practice of medicine, but it is expected that the physician is well-informed about the product and that the "off-label" use is based on sound scientific rationale and adequate medical evidence (29).

Several states in the United States (to date, Nevada, Oregon, Kansas, and Nebraska) have established restrictions or considered bans on solutions with PC/DC or DC until there is rigorous safety and efficacy data meeting standards set forth by the FDA. It is unknown but likely that other states will follow these restrictions.

Mesotherapy formulations, in contrast, may contain some FDA-approved medications for subcutaneous injection, such as hyaluronidase, lidocaine, and isoproterenol. These ingredients are not, however, approved distinctly for direct subcutaneous injection for the intent treatment of fat and/or cellulite (26).

CURRENT STATE OF KNOWLEDGE

Mechanism of Action

Early publications describing injection lipolysis suggest that PC, a phospholipid, was the major active ingredient in the formulation (3,5). As intravenous Lipostabil lowers blood lipids, it was initially assumed that PC's effect on fat *in serum* could explain why localized fat loss is observed after subcutaneous injection. Therefore, it was conjectured that PC could act in several ways, which included inducing a cascade of intracellular signaling leading to lipolysis, directly lysing fat cell membranes, or facilitating transit of triglycerides across cell membranes. These mechanisms are distinct from Lipostabil's capacity to pharmacologically induce changes in serum cholesterol and lipids. An unexpected discovery, initially held suspect by some, appears now to be a rational explanation why this formulation acts the way it does when injected subcutaneously.

The unexpected finding revealed that isolated DC, the other major component of *all* PC formulations (compounded or Lipostabil), causes significant cell death and cell lysis in keratinocyte cell cultures and extracted (ex vivo) porcine fat (Fig. 6.2) (30). Moreover, the addition of PC to DC has negligible effects on the activity of the formulation that could account for any significant activity. Schuller-Petrovic and colleagues (31) recently replicated these findings by performing similar studies in living tissue (Fig. 6.3). What this means is that reduction of fat at the sites of PC/DC injections appears to be due to rupturing of fat cell membranes by DC alone (30). It also means that DC could be effective as the sole agent in injection lipolysis. This was proven beyond doubt when studies revealed that human lipomas (18), and

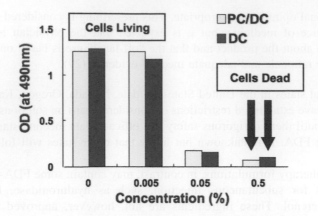

Figure 6.2 MTS cell viability assay measuring living keratinocytes exposed to phosphatidylcholine/deoxycholate (PC/DC) and deoxycholate (DC). Absorbance (OD) is directly related to cell viability. Increasing concentration of either PC/DC or DC alone augments cell death. Inclusion of PC in the PC/DC formulation has minimal effect compared to utilizing DC alone. *Source*: From Ref. 2, modified with permission.

abdominal (13), upper thigh (6), and submental fat (32), are reduced after DC injections (Figs. 6.4 and 6.5).

Furthermore, there are currently no experimental or clinical studies on adipose tissue investigating the effect of PC as an adipolytic, apoptotic, or detergent agent in isolation from DC. The research is limited in part because PC is insoluble in water. To perform studies on fat, PC requires a solvent to dissolve it in an aqueous solution. However, PC solvents such as DC, another bile salt, or even ethanol would similarly produce cell lysis and confound the results (30). It is generally agreed that PC's role in the Lipodissolve formulation as a lipolytic agent appears to be only speculative.

Although the definitive role of PC is unclear, it appears in one recent investigation that PC may decrease the severity of the posttreatment adverse reactions. Salti and colleagues (6) injected the upper thighs of 37 women with PC/DC into one hip and DC into the contralateral side. After four injection sessions spaced two months apart, they found that 90% of the patients responded. There were no significant differences in efficacy between the formulations, as both groups experienced similar reductions in upper thigh measurements (7%) and ultrasonically confirmed subcutaneous fat thickness (40%). The PC-containing formulation, however, caused less pain, bruising, swelling, and nodularity than the DC-treated side. Accounting for dilution, the DC content was 1.25% in the PC/DC formulation and 1.19% in the DC-only formulation. PC was suggested to somehow "emulsify" and remove fat destroyed by DC at the treatment site. Whether this proves consistent in additional studies remains to be seen, as these data contrast to a recently completed, exploratory, double-blind clinical trial utilizing injections of

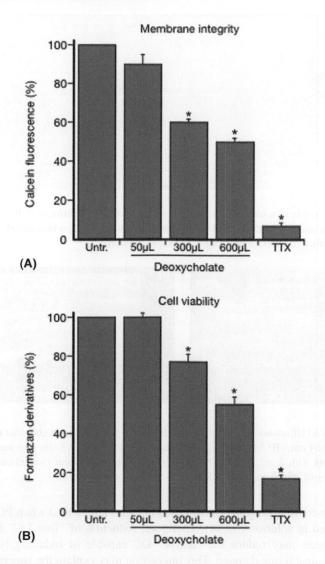

Figure 6.3 Effects of DC (2.5%) on rat fat cell membrane integrity (**A**) and cell viability (**B**) after repetitive dosing. The effects were observed 30 days following the application of 50, 300, or 600 µL of DC on Days 0, 7, and 28. Triton (TTX) 0.5% served as positive control. *Source*: From Ref. 31, reproduced with permission.

up to 2 mL of either DC (1%) or PC (5%)/DC(4.75%) into the submental fat (32). In this report, there were no obvious differences between treatment groups in the nature, intensity, or duration of adverse events, suggesting that under the study conditions PC did not reduce the severity or duration of adverse effects.

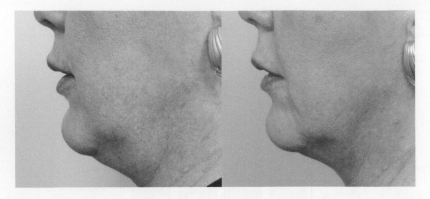

Figure 6.4 Profile of a woman before (*left*) and after (*right*) treatment of her submental fat with subcutaneous injections of 1% DC. Photographs were taken two months after five separate monthly treatments utilizing 1.0 mL per session.

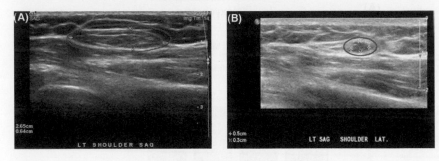

Figure 6.5 (**A**) Ultrasonic sagittal view of a lipoma in a patient's left shoulder measuring 2.65 cm × 0.64 cm. (**B**) Identical lipoma measuring 0.5 cm × 0.3 cm, two months after two treatments with 2 mL of 1% DC per session. Note echolucent (*white*) capsule surrounding lipoma, which was not palpable on physical examination.

Microscopic aggregates called *mixed micelles* are formed when PC and DC are combined in solution (33,34). Therefore, reduction of "free DC" by PC in these aggregate may reduce the "active" DC capable of inducing lysis, thus buffering against tissue damage. This interaction may explain the superior safety profile of the PC-containing formulation described in the preceding paragraph despite its almost equivalent DC concentration (1.25% vs. 1.19% DC). Along the same vein, the already low DC concentration (1%) in the submental trial revealed a more or less equal safety profile to the higher DC concentration (4.75%) formulation, perhaps due to "buffering" of PC. This speculation begs clarification with additional investigation. Although the phospholipid may reduce the morbidity of injection lipolysis treatment when equal concentrations of DC are used, decreasing DC concentration or adding lidocaine or even triamcinolone to the solution appears to be alternative approaches as well.

Deoxycholate

Deoxycholic acid, that is deoxycholate (Fig. 6.6), is a component of bile produced by intestinal bacteria after the release of primary bile acids (i.e., cholic acid) in the liver (35). Bile acids, which are stored in the gall bladder and secreted into the duodenum, consist of free and conjugated bile acids, which solubilize dietary fat. Most (90%–95%) DC is subsequently reabsorbed; excreted DC is replaced by ab initio synthesis from cholesterol in the liver. As bile acids are end products of cholesterol, they are not degraded into other catabolites. Approximately 1 g of DC is present at any time in an adult human, and it remains confined mostly to the enterohepatic circulation. Any DC present in the peripheral blood (normally approximately 0.56 μmol/L) can become elevated in certain liver conditions or post-operatively (35).

The use of bile salts (i.e., sodium deoxycholate) for experimental or medicinal purposes is not novel and has served numerous roles in science for decades. DC and other bile salts have been utilized to lyse and isolate the components of cell membranes (i.e., protein channels). It is also a common practice to incorporate them in intravenous formulations as physiologically compatible solvents in medications like Amphocin® (Pfizer), the common flu vaccine, and, of course, Lipostabil (36).

The effect of DC on tissue is profound. Animal and human tissues exposed to DC demonstrate hemorrhage, inflammation, and tissue necrosis (Fig. 6.7). By acting like a nonionic detergent, DC induces pores in cell membranes (33), thus causing leaking of cytoplasm contents and destabilizing and lysing of cellular membranes. This accounts for the localized inflammation (erythema, swelling, and tenderness) and essentially controlled injury at the sites of injection.

Few areas in aesthetic medicine are as exciting as minimally invasive fat loss. Introducing injection lipolysis into a practice can become an exciting endeavor, yet an appreciation for the aforementioned (scientific and theoretically based) discussion will bear relevance to the practice and evolution of this technique.

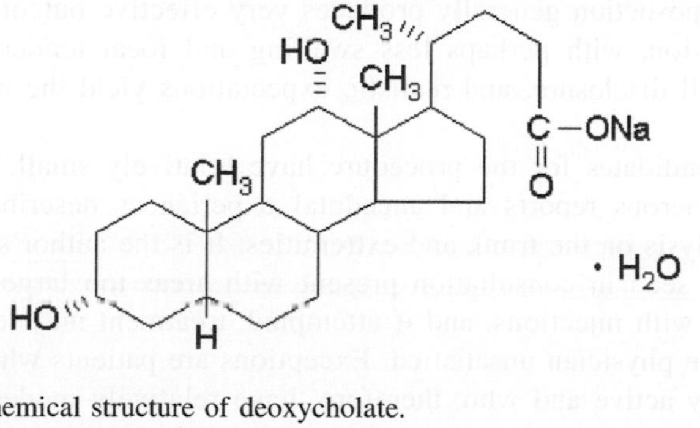

Figure 6.6 Chemical structure of deoxycholate.

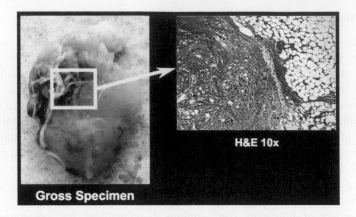

Figure 6.7   Excised lipoma two days after injection with sodium deoxycholate (1%) revealing a well-demarcated area of hemorrhage grossly that corresponded microscopically to acute inflammation, extravasation of erythrocytes, and necrosis (hematoxylin and eosin, original magnification 10×). *Source*: From Ref. 2, modified with permission.

SETTING EXPECTATIONS, PATIENT SELECTION AND CLINICAL EXAMINATION

It is prudent to begin this section with a reality check—*injection lipolysis will not replace liposuction or weight loss as effective means to reduce body fat*. At this point in time, it is unrealistic to expect that any minimally invasive (i.e., nonsurgical) body shaping technology will replace liposuction anytime in the near future. Specifically, patients undergoing injection lipolysis should anticipate specific localized reactions and not liposuction-like fat volume reductions and dramatic contour improvement. Fat reduced with injection lipolysis is significantly less compared to liposuction; as well, multiple sessions producing localized tenderness and swelling are commonplace and may in fact be required for efficacy. These less than desirable symptoms persist most significantly several days postinjection and gradually regress over several weeks. In contrast, liposuction generally produces very effective outcomes after one treatment session, with perhaps less swelling and focal tenderness. Candid discussion, full disclosure, and realistic expectations yield the most satisfied patients.

Ideal candidates for the procedure have relatively small, localized fat deposits. Numerous reports and anecdotal experiences describe the use of injection lipolysis on the trunk and extremities. It is the author's opinion that most patients seen in consultation present with areas too large to be effectively treated with injections, and if attempted, treatment may leave both the patient and the physician unsatisfied. Exceptions are patients who are very fit and physically active and who, therefore, have relatively modest collections of fat on the hips, anterior abdomen, and bra-strap (inferolateral scapula) regions. Another consideration is that greater surface areas on the trunk may predispose patients to more significant adverse reactions (systemic and local). On the other hand, post-liposuction contour defects or only modest fat collections in sites too small for liposuction adequately respond to injection lipolysis.

The treatment area should ideally be approximately one inch in subcutaneous fat thickness upon pinching. Some of the most gratifying outcomes are observed in the submental (neck fat) region. The discussion hereafter focuses especially with this in mind.

Treatment sites should not reveal any significant skin laxity, or in the neck, platysmal banding. Postpartum skin laxity is apparently tightened after injection lipolysis (12), perhaps a testament to the profibrotic response of the treatment. Yet, in the author's experience, this is not significant effect clinically and should be reserved for cases where the patient prefers no other alternative (i.e., radiofrequency or surgical intervention). Patients at least 18 to approximately 50 years of age are generally best candidates. The patient should have maintained a stable body weight for the last six months (i.e., within 5% of the initial consultation weight).

Female patients who are pregnant, breast-feeding, or those of childbearing potential who are not observing adequate contraceptive precautions should not receive treatment. Laboratory studies are generally not necessary unless the patient reports a comorbid medical condition during the initial screening. Patients should therefore have normal blood counts, serum lipids, and liver and renal function. Darkly pigmented patients (skin types Fitzpatrick IV–VI) are at an increased risk for postinflammatory hyperpigmentation.

At the initial consultation, the patient must comprehend that swelling, local tenderness, and nodularity are anticipated *and necessary* for efficacy. Further, the patient should be explained that *multiple treatments (3–4) are necessary* to appreciate any changes in fat volume. Without adequate understanding of these basic principles, patients will become frustrated with the initial postinjection site reaction and discontinue treatment. The caveat is that in some patients, results can be felt after the first treatment once the healing takes place and inflammation subsides (2–3 weeks), but it is generally a good practice policy to underpromise and overdeliver.

Patients often inquire whether the fat-reducing effects are "permanent." Just as liposuction-aspirated fat will not recur, "chemically ablated" fat cells will not reappear. Yet, both of these techniques do not completely eliminate all the subcutaneous fat in the target areas; therefore, fat may return with gained bodyweight.

Pre- and posttreatment photography, examination, and subjective feedback are used to assess results, as photography alone cannot convey the "firmer, tighter" sensation most patients experience after treatment. Nonetheless, comparing standardized photographs of pre- and posttreatment profiles with patients is a useful and gratifying exercise.

TREATMENT

Submental Fat

Depending upon the patient's distribution of fat, treatment can be limited to the submental region or extended to include the mandible and jowls. Treatment along the lateral edge of the mandible can yield a pleasing enhancement to the jaw line contour and prominence. Combination treatment using injection lipolysis to the face and neck along with botulinum toxin to the masseter muscle, and tissue tightening using radiofrequency can provide dramatic facial contouring. Deep injections into tissue other than fat should be avoided. This can be adequately ensured by pinching the area prior to injection.

Truncal and Extremity Fat

Anterior abdomen, waistline (love handles), hips (upper lateral thighs), inferolateral scapula fat ("bra-fat"), and posterior upper arm fat are commonly treated. General approach to treatment is similar to submental fat, with the key principle is to ensure modest fat collections in physically fit patients and realistic expectations of mild-to-moderate improvements in the volume of fat in these larger regions.

Pretreatment is generally not necessary for any site. As a precaution against bruising, some physicians employ oral Arnica several days before the procedure, which is continued for several days afterward. A rapid prednisolone taper and high-dose acetaminophen may be initiated a day prior to the procedure to reduce swelling and tenderness.

Materials required for the procedure are listed in Table 6.1. DC and lidocaine in 3:1 ratio are drawn into the same syringe (e.g., 3.75 mL of DC is mixed with 1.25 mL of lidocaine for a total volume 5.0 mL). A white precipitate may become evident transiently as DC is mixed with lidocaine, but it should resolubilize spontaneously or with a gentle mix of the syringe. It is not advised to order premixed lidocaine and DC, as the stability of these solutions is not known. Optionally, triamcinolone may be mixed within the aforementioned solution. To date, there are no published studies and only anecdotal evidence to suggest that the steroid can have a profound effect on reducing the magnitude of localized

Table 6.1 Materials Required for Injection Lipolysis

30-gauge, 0.5-in. needles and 18-gauge, 1-in. needles for withdrawing medication
Depending on the total volume required, several 1-, 3-, or 5-mL syringes
Surgical marker or eyeliner pencil for mapping of injection sites
Isopropyl alcohol with cotton/gauze
Sodium deoxycholate (DC) at 1% (10 mg/mL) in sterile water (i.e., water for injection
    with 0.9% benzyl alcohol)
Lidocaine (1%) without epinephrine
Optional: triamcinolone (10 mg/mL)

---

reactions. To this end, 0.25 mL of triamcinolone acetonide (10 mg/mL) is mixed with 1.0 mL lidocaine and 3.75 DC to yield a 0.05% (0.5 mg/mL) solution of the steroid. Injection directly into the fat and its wide distribution in the treatment area will reduce the risk of dermal atrophy and subcutaneous irregularities. It should be kept in mind that the total systemic dose of triamcinolone may be significant if large areas are being treated and, in such instances, the agent should be avoided or diluted further.

Patients are made comfortable either sitting upright or lying down and the treatment site is exposed, cleansed with alcohol, and delineated by placing marks in a staggered manner, 1.5 cm apart (Fig. 6.8). Nonfacial injections appear to be

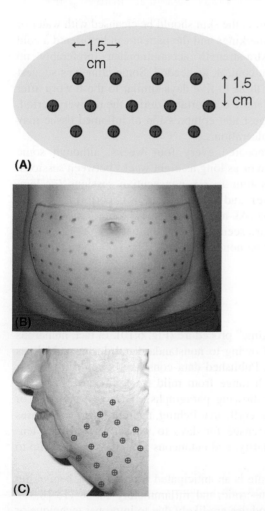

(A)

(B)

(C)

Figure 6.8 (A) Illustrative placement of each 0.25- to 0.33-mL injection in a staggered manner 1.5 cm apart from one another. (B) Abdomen and (C) submental areas marked accordingly.

less painful, so topical anesthesia is usually not needed but may be offered. Injections of 0.25 to 0.33 mL are made into the *mid-subcutaneous fat* to circumvent migration of the solution into the dermis and the muscle fascia. The needle is withdrawn without pressure on the syringe plunger to avoid leakage of the detergent into the dermis (which can induce necrosis). The needle is subsequently moved to the next site and the process is repeated (Fig. 6.9).

The skin may be pinched for more accurate—and, therefore, safer—placement of the solution in thinner areas (i.e., submental area, triceps). Total volume injected per session is site-dependent. Typical injected volumes vary from 2 to 5 mL for relatively small submental fat collections to 20 mL in the hips, waist, or abdomen.

Immediately after the procedure, the skin should be cleansed with water or alcohol to remove blood and skin markings and the patient can be offered a cold pack for increased comfort. Extra-strength acetaminophen (preferably no NSAIDs) is recommended for pain control, as needed. Some clinicians suggest compression garments be used for three to five days similar to those worn after liposuction. Patients are reportedly more comfortable during the recovery period, but there is some evidence to suggest that compression of inflamed tissue may predispose some patients to skin ulceration.

Treatments are typically repeated every four weeks, although some authors recommend as short as two or as long as eight weeks between sessions. A standard treatment regimen is four to six consecutive sessions (or less, depending upon patient's response), and final evaluation is performed two to three months after the last session. As noted previously, three treatments are generally required before results are seen or felt by the patient; the risk of not explaining this to the patient may be noncompliance, disappointment, and loss to follow-up.

ADVERSE EFFECTS

Injection lipolysis is not a "lunch-time" procedure (Fig. 6.10). In fact, numerous complications have been reported owing to nonstandardized dosing guidelines and improper injection technique. Published data consistently confirm predictable posttreatment sequelae, which range from mild to significant in severity (detailed chronologically in the following paragraphs). The most common of these effects are immediate edema, erythema, itching, and burning; ecchymoses and significant swelling typically ensue for days to weeks; and residual tenderness, hyperpigmentation, nodularity, and cutaneous numbness may last up to a month or longer.

Nodularity at the treatment site is an anticipated reaction. This benign but unsettling finding is a focus of necrotic and inflammatory tissue (13,18,31). Anecdotal reports of unresolved nodules are likely due to improper technique or use of high-concentration DC (>2.5%) in isolation.

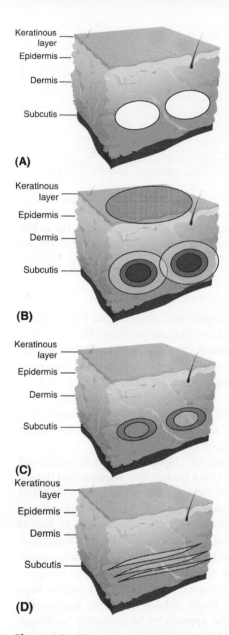

Figure 6.9 Illustrative chronological sequence of changes in subcutaneous tissue in cross section after injection with detergent. Medication is placed in relative close approximation (1.5 cm) directly within the subcutaneous fat so as to reduce the irregularities (**A**). Intense inflammation and cutaneous erythema (**B**) occur within 24 hours. Nodule (**C**) develops at the focus of ablated fat and healing tissue within several weeks. Fibrosis and volume reduction (**D**) develop after several months.

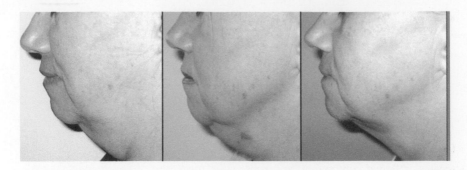

Figure 6.10 Profile of a woman before (*far left image*) and after (*far right image*) treatment of her submental fat with subcutaneous injections of 10 mL of 1% DC and 1% lidocaine (7.5-mL DC and 2.25-mL lidocaine) monthly for four months. The middle image was taken 24 hours after second injection session, revealing significant edema and areas of ecchymoses.

Gastrointestinal symptoms, such as nausea and diarrhea, are likely related to a bolus systemic effect from PC or DC. Less frequent adverse effects, such as light-headedness and intermenstrual bleeding, have been reported with high doses of PC/DC combinations (6,10,12), leading some authors to recommend maximum doses of 2.5 g of PC per injection session (or 2250 mg DC for a 4.5% formulation of DC) (12). A very conservative dilution (1% DC) and doses up to 20 mL per session using the protocol and materials described in this chapter will yield the relatively low dose of 150 mg DC and no PC. As a reminder, the human body normally contains approximately 1 g of DC.

Aside from total volume or dose injected, injection depth is considered one of the most critical safety issues (12). There is currently unpublished data to suggest that DC has some *relative* specificity to fat; nevertheless, published data demonstrates that haphazard or inadvertent injection deep into muscle or superficially into the dermis may induce necrosis. Concentrations as low as 0.5% DC (in exclusion of PC) (13), as well as the standard Lipodissolve concentrations of PC/DC, have revealed muscle and vascular necrosis microscopically (30). Although these findings have not clinically translated to rampant, morbid complications, accounts of skin ulceration (10,22–24,37) and perhaps the high incidence of ecchymoses are likely related to these nonspecific detergent effects on tissue. Skin ulceration appears to be primarily technique dependent. Concentration of detergent is also a factor, but conservative dilution (approximately 1% DC) is a further safeguard. Skin ulceration is not unheard of during sclerotherapy, especially following extravascular injection of the sclerosing solution (38). As with other injectables, proper technique, training, and clinical experience will help to avert undesirable effects and confer a superior outcome.

Further Considerations

Ulceration, scarring, contour irregularities or skin indentation, hyperpigmentation, superficial infections (including atypical mycobacteria), gastrointestinal effects, and liver failure have been reported anecdotally in the popular press and on the Internet (22–25). A reasonable conclusion based solely on these sources of information would be that injection lipolysis is inherently unsafe and outrightly dangerous despite the training and experience of the injecting clinician and regardless of the source of the medication. However, the generally safe outcomes reported in peer-reviewed literature and anecdotal experience among many clinicians suggest otherwise. It is likely that most of these deleterious outcomes are a direct consequence of failing to adhere to aseptic injection technique and improper placement of the medication. The mantra "too much, too close, too high" refers to avoiding injecting more than 0.4 mL of solution per site, placing the injections too superficially (intradermally or higher), and injecting sites too close to one another (<1.5 cm).

A report by Davis and colleagues (37) describes an unfortunate case of "mesotherapy-induced noninfectious granulomatous panniculitis" in a young woman injected with DC by a nurse in a home office for the purposes of reducing cellulite. Violaceous nodules and erosions on the thighs, buttocks, knees, and lower legs were evident on examination. The injection technique, DC concentration, and the volume injected were unknown. Apparent from the accompanying photographs, in addition to the unorthodox sites (knees, ankles, popliteal fossae), was the haphazard, closely spaced distribution of the lesions. These outcomes are a testament to the aggressive nature of treatment by poorly trained practitioners. It is worth keeping in mind that the literature supports safety and efficacy with a measured and conservative approach, worth repeating here: small (0.2–0.4 mL) aliquots of solution containing 1% DC (alone) or 4.2% to 4.7% DC (with 5% PC) spaced at least 1.5 cm apart and directed into the subcutaneous fat.

The long- and short-term local and systemic effects of these medications in larger populations are not known since they have not been rigorously studied in controlled FDA trials. In light of relative easy access to appealing "fat-dissolving" injections and the lack of regulations, sustained use by practitioners without proper training or supporting data may expose patients to additional, so far unknown, risks. As of this writing, Kythera Biopharmaceuticals (Calabasas, CA) is conducting phase II FDA trials with a detergent-based lipolytic medication for both aesthetic and nonaesthetic indications (39).

Another consideration is the eventual fate of ablated adipocytes. The majority (>75%) of the adipocyte volume is triglycerides (40). Lipid-laden macrophages and an intense lymphomononuclear infiltrate are evident within injected fat (13,14,18,41,42). Several hypotheses have been generated by reviewing the sequence of events that occur in adipose tissue after blunt trauma (40): (*i*) released triglycerides from ablated cell membranes are likely processed by lipoprotein lipases on extracellular membranes to glycerol and free fatty acids; (*ii*) water-soluble components of triglycerides (glycerol) are transported to the liver via the serum; (*iii*) the fat-soluble components of triglycerides (free fatty acids) bind to albumin and are metabolized by organs; and (*iv*) cellular debris are engulfed by macrophages and carried away via the lymphatics into the general circulation and metabolized by the liver.

As of this writing, laboratory testing in humans treated with PC/DC (11) and DC (13) does not suggest any significant alterations in blood lipids, nor any other chemistry or blood counts. A lipid profile (total lipids, triglyceride, and cholesterol) two hours, one day, and two, four, six, eight weeks, and six months after an abdominal treatment using 10 mL of 1.25% or 0.5% DC (totaling 125 mg and 50 mg of DC, respectively) was normal at all times in all subjects (13). In light of the relatively small volumes of the injected detergent and correspondingly modest areas of treated fat, combined with slow (i.e., weeks to months) resolution of inflammation (13), it is unlikely that conservative (i.e. <20 mL per session) injectable lipolysis treatment would lead to acute fatty liver in healthy patients; however, a definitive confirmation is essential. In comparison, rigorous studies have neither revealed fatty infiltration of the liver nor any augmentation of blood lipids after the novel ablative, minimally invasive, high-frequency ultrasound treatments (43,44).

The adverse events described in sections "Local Reactions" and "Systemic Reactions" are a sequence of the anticipated reactions, and therefore should be explained thoroughly to the patient. Patients who may be accustomed to the relatively benign localized reactions of injectable fillers and botulinum toxin would likely benefit from this explanation. In addition, a reassuring call to patients the next day is, in my experience, a very good practice.

Local Reactions

Immediately After Injection to Day 1

Most patients experience mild tenderness, burning, or itching despite lidocaine. Erythema and moderate edema will persist.

Days 2 to 3

Edema will be moderate to significant, as will focal tenderness and ecchymoses, although erythema will have resolved (Fig. 6.10). Swelling is often described as "jelly-like" by patients. The majority of swelling subsides after 3 days. Cutaneous anesthesia may begin and persist for 1 to 2 weeks. Similar to other injectables, bruising may take a week to resolve. Initial treatment is best performed immediately before a weekend when no social activity is planned. After this, patients will anticipate their reaction and adjust their work and social schedule accordingly. Interestingly, most patients report a significantly less robust inflammatory reaction after subsequent treatments, even with similar volumes.

Day 3 to Week 1

Tenderness and edema slowly resolve, but may persist to a milder degree, along with superficial paresthesia (mild numbness, not tingling) beyond this period.

Weeks 2 to 4

Most anticipated adverse events have passed, although firm, minimally tender subcutaneous nodules may be felt at sporadic injection sites. Superficial anesthesia is common as well, but will resolve in this period of time. Patients should be reassured that the nodules are ablated fat and a sign of the effectiveness of treatment, and that these non-apparent areas will continue to resolve as the site recovers. Nodules, if present at follow-up, should not be injected directly, lending additional support for pinching the skin prior to injection.

Week 4 and Ahead

Rarely, localized nodularity persists beyond four to six weeks.

Anecdotal observation suggests that the inclusion of triamcinolone in the formulation may attenuate edema and tenderness. The incidence of nodularity, however, does not appear to be significantly affected.

Systemic Reactions

Gastrointestinal effects, such as nausea and diarrhea, several hours to several days after treatment have been described by some authors following the use of Lipodissolve (PC/DC) (6,12) as well as DC alone (6). It is therefore prudent to limit total volume to 20 mL (or 150 mg DC total) per injection session. Published and ongoing studies with DC reveal no systemic alterations in serum chemistries, lipids, or blood counts at conservative doses.

CONCLUSIONS

With rigorous study of its safety and efficacy in large, diverse populations, injection lipolysis and perhaps other non-ablative mesotherapy ingredients may eventually become an acceptable minimally invasive injectable therapy for fat. For patients unwilling to have liposuction, those with collections of fat too modest for liposuction, or those with postliposuction irregularities, this procedure may add to the increasing—and exciting—number of modalities on the next frontier of aesthetic medicine.

Despite the controversy and even skepticism over its efficacy, injectable lipolytic treatments are here to stay. Mandatory and extensive safety testing and numerous clinical trials will be required for regulatory approval. Until then, physicians interested in this technique should seek training and become very familiar with the literature in order to deliver a relatively safe, effective, and gratifying procedure to their properly selected patients.

REFERENCES

1. Wanner M, Avram M. An evidence-based assessment of treatments for cellulite. J Drugs Dermatol 2008; 7:341–345.
2. Rotunda AM, Kolodney MS. Mesotherapy and phosphatidylcholine injections: historical clarification and review. Dermatol Surg 2006; 32:465–480.
3. Rittes PG. The use of phosphatidylcholine for correction of lower lid bulging due to prominent fat pads. Dermatol Surg 2001; 27:391–392.
4. Treacy P, Goldberg D. Use of phosphatidylcholine for the correction of lower lid bulging due to prominent fat pads. J Cosmet Laser Ther 2006; 8:129–132.
5. Ablon G, Rotunda AM. Treatment of lower eyelid fat pads using phosphatidylcholine: clinical trial and review. Dermatol Surg 2004; 30:422–427.
6. Salti G, Ghersetich I, Tantussi F, et al. Phosphatidylcholine and sodium deoxycholate in the treatment of localized fat: a double-blind, randomized study. Dermatol Surg 2008; 34:60–66.
7. Rittes PG. Complications of Lipostabil Endova for treating localized fat deposits. Aesthet Surg J 2007; 27:146–149.
8. Rullan PP, Hexsel D. Phosphatidylcholine injections for lipolysis of neck and jowls—50 case presentation. Presented at the 2005 Annual Meeting of the American Society of Dermatologic Surgery/American College of Mohs Micrographic Surgery and Cutaneous Oncology Combined Annual Meeting, October 27–31, 2005. Atlanta, GA.
9. Hexsel DM, Serra M, de Oliveira Dal'Forno T, et al. Cosmetic uses of injectable PC on the face. Otolarngol Clin N Am 2005; 38:1119–1129.
10. Palmer M, Curran J, Bowler P. Clinical experience and safety using phosphatidylcholine injections for the localized reduction of subcutaneous fat: a multicentre, retrospective UK study. J Cosmet Dermatol 2006; 5:218–226.
11. Hexsel DM, Serra M, de Oliveira Dal'Forno T, et al. Phosphatidylcholine in the treatment of localized fat. J Drugs Dermatol 2003; 2:511–518.
12. Duncan D. Lipodissolve for subcutaneous fat reduction and skin retraction. Aesthet Surg J 2005; 25:530–543.
13. Yagina Odo YME, Cuce LC, Odo LM, et al. Action of sodium deoxycholate on subcutaneous human tissue: local and systemic effects. Dermatol Surg 2007; 33: 178–188.
14. Bechara FG, Sand M, Hoffmann K, et al. Fat tissue after lipolysis of lipomas: a histopathological and immunohistochemical study. J Cutan Pathol 2007; 34: 552–557.
15. Kopera D, Binder B, Toplak H. Intralesional lipolysis with phosphatidylcholine for the treatment of lipomas: pilot study. Arch Dermatol 2006; 142:395–396.
16. Rittes PG. The use of phosphatidylcholine for correction of localized fat deposits. Aesthetic Plast Surg 2003; 27:315–318.
17. Myers P. The cosmetic use of phosphatidylcholine in the treatment of localized fat deposits. Cosmet Dermatol 2006;19:4160–4120.
18. Rotunda AM, Ablon G, Kolodney MS. Lipomas treated with subcutaneous deoxycholate injections. J Am Acad Dermatol 2005; 53:973–978.
19. Consumer Safety Alert on Fat Dissolving Injections. Oct 8, 2007. Available at: http://www.prnewswire.com/. Accessed May 28, 2011.

20. American Society for Dermatologic Surgery. Emerging technology report: mesotherapy. Available at: http://www.asds-net.org/Media/PositionStatements/emerging_technology-mesotherapy.html. Accessed May 28, 2011.
21. American Society for Aesthetic Plastic Surgery. American Society for Aesthetic Plastic Surgery warns patients to steer clear of injection fat loss treatments. May 14, 2007. Available at: http://www.surgery.org/press/news-release.php?iid=475. Accessed May 28, 2011.
22. Rundle RL. Popular treatment that aims to melt fat draws scrutiny. Wall Street Journal. June 12, 2007. Available at: http://online.wsj.com/article/SB118160554567831887.html?mod=home_health_right. Accessed May 28, 2011.
23. Boodman SG. Can Shots Safely 'Melt Away Fat'? Washington Post. Tuesday, June 26, 2007. Available at: http://www.washingtonpost.com/wp-dyn/content/article/2007/06/22/AR2007062201870.html. Accessed May 28, 2011.
24. Walsh N. Some would halt lipolysis tx pending safety data. Skin Allergy News 2004; 25:26.
25. Available at http://www.lipotreatmentfacts.org/. Accessed July 25, 2011.
26. Rotunda AM, Avram MM, Avram AS. Cellulite: is there a role for injectables? J Cosmet Laser Ther 2005; 7:147–154.
27. Caruso MK, Roberts AT, Bissoon L, et al. An evaluation of mesotherapy solutions for inducing lipolysis and treating cellulite. J Plast Reconstr Aesthet Surg 2008; 61:1321–1324.
28. Greenway FL, Bray GA. Regional fat loss from the thigh in obese women after adrenergic modulation. Clin Ther 1987; 9:663–669.
29. United States Food and Drug Administration (USFDA). Statement on Lipo-Dissolve. February 2, 2008. Available at: http://www.fda.gov. Accessed May 28, 2011.
30. Rotunda AM, Suzuki H, Moy RL, et al. Detergent effects of sodium deoxycholate are a major feature of an injectable phosphatidylcholine formulation used for localized fat dissolution. Dermatol Surg 2004; 30:1001–1008.
31. Schuller-Petrovic S, Wölkart G, Höfler G, et al. Tissue-toxic effects of phosphatidylcholine/deoxycholate after subcutaneous injection for fat dissolution in rats and a human volunteer. Dermatol Surg 2008; 34:529–534.
32. Rotunda AM, Weiss SR, Rivkin LS. Randomized, double-blind clinical trial of subcutaneously injected deoxycholate versus a phosphatidylcholine/deoxycholate combination for the reduction of submental fat. Dermatol Surg 2009; 35:792–803.
33. Jones MN. Surfactants in membrane solubilisation. Int J Pharm 1999; 177:137–159.
34. Bangham JA, Lea EJ. The interaction of detergents with bilayer lipid membranes. Biochim Biophys Acta 1978; 511:388–396.
35. Bahar RJ. Bile acid transport. Gastroenterol Clin North Am 1999; 28:27–58.
36. Dürr M, Hager J, Löhr JP. Investigations on mixed micelle and liposome preparations for parenteral use based on soya phosphatidylcholine. Eur J Biopharma 1994; 40:147–156.
37. Davis MD, Wright TI, Shehan JM. A complication of mesotherapy: noninfectious granulomatous panniculitis. Arch Dermatol 2008; 144:808–809.
38. Goldman MP, Sadick NS, Weiss RA. Cutaneous necrosis, telangiectatic matting, and hyperpigmentation following sclerotherapy. Etiology, prevention, and treatment. Dermatol Surg 1995; 21:19–29.
39. Available at: http://www.kytherabiopharma.com/. Accessed July 25, 2011.

40. Spencer B. What Happens to the Fat After Treatment With the UltraShape Device [Ph.D. thesis]. Available at: http://www.ultrashape.com. Accessed May 28, 2011.

41. Rose PT, Morgan M. Histological changes associated with mesotherapy for fat dissolution. J Cosmet Laser Ther 2005; 7:17–19.

42. Salles AG, Valler CS, Ferreira MC. Histologic response to injected phosphatidylcholine in fat tissue: experimental study in a new rabbit model. Aesthetic Plast Surg 2006; 30:479–484.

43. Garcia-Murray E, Rivas OA, Stecco K, et al. Evaluation of the acute and chronic systemic and metabolic effects from the use of high intensity focused ultrasound for adipose tissue removal and non-invasive body sculpting. American Society of Plastic Surgeons, 2005 Annual Meeting, E-Poster Session.

44. Fodor PB, Smoller BR, Stecco KA, et al. Biochemical changes in adipocytes and lipid metabolism secondary to the use of high-intensity focused ultrasound for non-invasive body sculpting. American Society of Aesthetic Plastic Surgery 2006 Annual Meeting, Poster Session.

7

Autologous fat transfer and other synthetic facial volumizers

Kimberly Butterwick

INTRODUCTION

Although autologous fat transfer (AFT) has been described in the literature for over 100 years, as a rejuvenating procedure it has waxed and waned in popularity. As recently as 20 years ago, the subject of facial volumizing was limited to a relatively small group of cosmetic surgeons advocating AFT for true facial rejuvenation. In this century, facial volume restoration with both AFT and synthetic fillers is enjoying a renaissance. Several trends have changed the landscape in the 21st century: an awareness that a rhytidectomy is not truly rejuvenating without volume replacement, an increasing demand by the public for non-invasive cosmetic procedures, and an increasing availability of synthetic products with consequent direct marketing to the public for facial volume restoration. Thus, not only have cosmetic surgeons revised their approach to rejuvenation, but the general public has also gained sophistication as well. Aging baby boomers remain in the competitive workforce for longer periods of time and desire discrete, natural outcomes and minimal downtimes. They want to avoid the overdone look of facial surgery as well as the prolonged recovery time. Consequently, in the United States, the number of nonsurgical procedures rose from approximately 1 million to more than 9 million from 1997 to 2005 (1). Soft tissue filler procedures increased 39% over the same period of time. Despite the slowing economy, the number of nonsurgical procedures rose to 10.4 million by 2008. Although AFT is nearly the ideal volumizer, having no allergenic potential, being readily available in most patients, and having an over 100-year track record of safety, it is still a more invasive procedure. On the other hand, newer synthetic fillers are threatening AFT as the preferred volumizer because of their ease of use, minimal downtime, and improved and predictable longevity.

This chapter explores the current state of AFT as well as the use of newer synthetic fillers currently available for correcting facial volume loss.

BACKGROUND

Before examining AFT and synthetic fillers, it is essential to understand the key role that volume loss plays in the aged appearance of the face. As recently as the 1980s, conventional wisdom among most cosmetic surgeons was that facial aging was the result of gravity-induced ptosis that could be remedied with rhytidectomy. However, it was noted by advocates of AFT that the laxity of aging skin was not a result of gravity, but largely because of loss of volume of underlying hard and soft tissue (2). They recognized the changing shape of the face as one ages, with the triangle of youth, having its base at the malar cheek and apex at the chin, replaced by an inverted triangle, with the base at the jowls and apex at the nose (Fig. 7.1). The aging face becomes a longer and narrower face. These changes occur as a result of atrophy of not only subcutaneous fat but also muscle and bone, with bone loss possibly of primary importance (3). Pessa and others have also shown remodeling of the bone with age, eventuating in a relatively larger orbit and a smaller maxilla (4–6). The maxilla not only shortens but also there is a posterior retrusion of the maxilla causing the platform for soft tissue to give way. CT scans have shown changes in key angles of the face and an enlargement of the pyriform aperture with age (7). The pyriform and maxillary angles become more acute over time, again reducing the forward projection of the face and the underlying support for soft tissue. The bony changes seem to have direct consequences in the aging face: as the orbit enlarges, the eyes become more hollow; as the maxilla shortens, the overlying soft tissue of

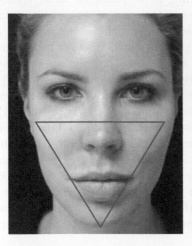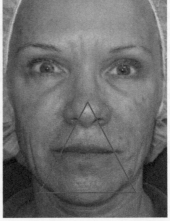

Figure 7.1 Changing facial shape from a youthful triangle, emphasizing the mid-face, to a widened lower face with an inverted triangle shape.

the mid-face flattens and falls. In addition, the mandible shrinks over time, causing a waviness of the lower third of the face and an apparent retraction of the chin (8). These hard tissue changes are further exacerbated by atrophy of the fat compartments of the face. It has been recognized for decades that facial fat atrophies over time. However, newer data from the study carried out by Rorich and Pessa have shown multiple discrete fat compartments of the face, demonstrated by injecting 30 fresh cadavers with methylene blue and observing the distribution over a 24-hour period (9). There is a large lateral cheek fat compartment that encompasses the temple and the entire lateral face and mandibular angle. When this area atrophies, the overlying skin collapses and becomes ptotic. This study also revealed several fat compartments of the mid-cheek that tend to shear and slide over time, causing accelerated deflation of fat. The facial muscles become lax with these hard and soft tissue changes and either hypertrophy—as in the case of the platysmal bands—or atrophy and fail to provide support for these compartments of fat. Although these studies are small and limited, they do underscore an increasing knowledge of structural changes with age, with findings in sharp contrast with previously held notions of aging. As more evidence accumulates, the need for full-face volumizing is fast approaching and even replacing more conventional methods for restoring youthful structure.

HISTORICAL PERSPECTIVE

Historically, AFT has been the only technique for full face volume restoration. This is a technique utilized since the late 1800s when Neuber (10) observed excellent aesthetic results after transferring multiple 1-cm fat grafts from the arm to fill facial depressions caused by tuberculosis. Other early reports followed, including that from Lexer who in 1909 treated facial atrophy by transferring fat from the abdomen to the malar infraorbital area (11). Upon histopathologic examination of transplanted fat, Tuffier noted in 1911 that a large percentage of fat was actually absorbed and replaced with fibrous tissue (12). In the same year, Bruning injected autologous fat for post-rhinoplasty deformities (13). A large gap in reported cases ensued until Peer, in the 1950s published studies on the retention of transplanted fat (14). He determined that eight months after transplantation, grafts appeared as normal adipose tissue microscopically, but lost approximately 45% of their weight and volume after one year because of absorption.

Another lull in the interest in AFT followed until the late 1970s and early 1980s, when an increase in the interest was directly fueled by advancements in liposuction by Illouz, as well as Fischer and Fischer (15,16). Fat grafting was still an open or semi-open procedure until Fournier's inadvertent discovery in 1985 that fat could be extracted with a syringe and needle (17). He named his technique "microlipoinjection," and expanded the popularity of AFT. This renewed interest prompted further inquiry into optimal techniques for harvesting, processing, and injection of fat for enhanced adipocyte survival and longevity of results. The literature of the 1980s abounds with anecdotal and empirical reports regarding fat cell viability, but there is an unfortunate lack of controlled studies. Not all reports were positive: some reported dissatisfaction with transient results (18).

The 1990s brought a second, even more explosive, surge of interest in liposuction, with an eightfold rise in the number of procedures performed in the United States from 1990 to 1999 (19). This boon was due in large part to Klein's introduction of the tumescent technique, allowing liposuction to be performed less invasively under local anesthesia with minimal postoperative downtime and unparalleled patient safety (20). Klein, a dermatologic surgeon, opened the door for more dermatologists to enter the arena of cosmetic surgery with a safe procedure that could be performed in the office. The increase in liposuction procedures naturally led to an increased interest in cosmetic uses for the removed fat, namely AFT, for filling of furrows and correction of soft tissue defects. A variety of improved techniques and strategies for AFT emerged.

Concepts regarding fat transfer changed during this period. One of the most significant changes in technique was a shift from overcorrecting in order to compensate for postprocedure fat loss to transferring small volumes of fat. This change reflected a transition in the concept of fat from a temporary resorbed filler to a living graft. In the 1980s and early 1990s, it was not uncommon for large volumes of fat to be placed with deforming overcorrection of 50% or more (21). Patients would experience embarrassing overcorrection for weeks. Adding insult to injury, the rate of resorption of these volumes was often variable, unpredictable, and asymmetric. In the late 1980s, Coleman championed the survival theory of fat grafting and developed a method he called Lipostructure^{TM} (22). He advocated placing small strands, or "parcels," of fat with repetitive passes into multiple new tissue planes, reasoning that a blood supply was more easily established. Gentle atraumatic handling of the fat cells was required for survival of the cells. Others reported improved longevity with injection of smaller volumes and less traumatic harvesting and processing (23,24). In 1994, Carpaneda validated these empiric findings with a histological study comparing the viability of fat cylinders of different diameters (25). He found that smaller fat grafts, less than 3 mm in diameter, had optimal viability. At two months, viable fat cells were noted only in the peripheral zone of larger grafts having diameters of 3.5 mm or greater. In a review of literature of the 1990s, small fat grafts versus overcorrection with a fat bolus was the common factor in studies reporting good longevity of fat (26).

The 1990s also ushered a change in the indications for fat transfer. In the 1980s, fat was typically indicated for deep rhytides of the nasolabial and marionette regions. The new 1990s concept was full-facial replacement of volume, not simply directed toward specific rhytids and furrows. It was increasingly recognized among aesthetic surgeons performing AFT that filling lines did not necessarily rejuvenate a patient's appearance. It was further realized by Berman,

Fournier and others that traditional approaches to ptotic skin with rhytidectomy or blepharoplasty, did not equate with a youthful appearance (27,28). They recognized the need to correct the atrophy of hard and soft tissues that occurs with age for a truly rejuvenated appearance with three-dimensional contour. To restore full-facial volume, larger quantities in the range of 20 to 100 ml or more were advocated. Guerrerosantos further pointed out that soft tissues may thin out even more after rhytidectomy, resulting in more rapid aging and a skeletonized appearance (29). Restoring volume to the aged face was thus first appreciated by those advocating panfacial volume restoration with AFT, as evidenced by the literature of the late 1990s and early 2000s (30,31).

These opinions were initially overlooked by the majority of plastic and cosmetic surgeons who preferred traditional surgery, as well as by most dermatologists who were accustomed to filling fine lines with bovine collagen. Panfacial filling with AFT was relegated to a relatively small group of aesthetic surgeons of various specialties. Although AFT was the natural choice for panfacial volumization, the invasiveness of the procedure, the downtime, and the reports of unpredictable results limited the popularity of the procedure. However, there were few alternatives for volume restoration as the 21st century began. Quantities of 10 ml or more were not feasible with the synthetic 1-ml dermal fillers of the 1990s (bovine collagen) primarily because of expense of numerous syringes and the temporary nature of those fillers. Silicon injections were practiced by some, but the filler was not FDA-approved. Safety and legal issues deterred most physicians.

Things have changed in the past decade. The ease and efficacy of neurotoxins for upper facial aging created a discrepancy with the aged lower face. Patients wanted a comparably simple solution for lower face wrinkles and the demand for noninvasive fillers grew exponentially (32). At the same time, newer synthetic fillers have been developed, which not only offer line filling but also have enough volume, bulk, and viscosity for structural volumizing with the minimal downtime that patients prefer. Direct marketing to consumers by the filler manufacturers have also fueled the demand for fillers. Aesthetic surgeons from many specialties have embraced the concept of full-face volumizing, and medical literature and lay magazines abound with articles on "volumizing" as if it were a new concept. Products currently utilized for volumizing in the United States are shown in Table 7.1. Although not FDA-approved specifically for volumizing, most agents are FDA-approved for filling of the nasolabial folds. Given the success of these fillers, even more volumizing filler products will be entering the market in the near future that will give the clinician even more choices. Because it still has certain advantages over synthetic fillers, AFT will most likely always remain an option, albeit a more invasive one. No matter what the filler agent, today's challenge is to volumize the face with an aesthetic eye, using adequate volumes while still controlling costs, maximizing longevity of results, and minimizing adverse effects.

Table 7.1 Injectable Dermal Fillers for Volumizing the Face

Category/Product	Treatment sessions	Duration
HA	1	
Restylane		6–12 months
Perlane		6–12 months
Juvederm		Up to 12 months
Juvederm Ultra Plus		
Prevelle Silk		
Hylaform		3–6 months
Hydrelle		
CaHA	1–2	
Radiesse		9–12 months
PLLA	2–5	
Sculptra		12–24 months
PMMA	2 or more	
Arte Fill		Permanent

HA, hyaluronic acid; CaHA, calcium hydroxylapatite; PLLA, poly-L-lactic acid; PMMA, polymethyl methacrylate.

CURRENT STATE OF KNOWLEDGE

Analysis of Volume Loss and Aesthetic Goals

When assessing a patient for volume loss, it is helpful to examine the face from three perspectives. The first is to look at the symmetry of the face as a whole utilizing classic proportions (33). Divide the face into the ideal proportion of horizontal thirds from the frontal hairline to glabella, glabella to subnasale, and subnasale to mentum (Fig. 7.2). The one-third/two-thirds ratio is also an ideal from the subnasale to lip to mentum. In addition, divide the face vertically into fifths, with the mid-face divided into five portions, each the width of one eye (Fig. 7.2). The physician can apply these divisions mentally or actually draw them on a photograph of the patient to help determine which areas are relatively deficient.

The second perspective is to assess each third of the face for specific areas of volume loss (Table 7.2). In the upper third, examine the shape of the forehead, whether it has full slightly rounded contour or a more slanted contour. Assess the glabella and nasal root for fullness versus a collapsed, concave appearance. Check for temporal hollowing and a deflated versus contoured brow. In the middle-third, assess the periorbital region, especially the lid-to-cheek transition that ideally is continuous but often interrupted by the nasojugal crease or tear trough. The lateral lid-to-cheek transition should be noted as well. The antero-medial and mid-cheek should be assessed for fullness. From a side view, the mid-cheek should project as far as a line drawn vertically from the cornea of the eye (5). Laterally, the malar and zygomaticotemporal regions should be

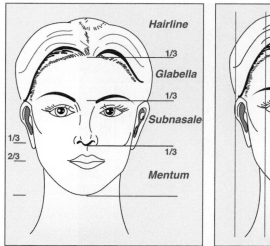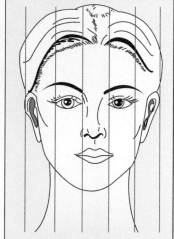

Figure 7.2 Ideal proportions applied to the patient's face to assess areas of deficit.

Table 7.2 Manifestations of Facial Volume Loss

Upper third
 Forehead—flat or slanted
 Glabella/nasal root—deflated, loss of light reflex
 Temporal hollowing
 Brow—flat, loss of contour
Middle third
 Loss of lid-cheek continuity
 Tear trough deformity
 Flattened mid-cheek, mid-cheek crease
 Bony prominences visible
 Malar descent
 Nasal tip descent
Lower Third
 Lengthening of upper lip
 Loss of lip projection
 Nasolabial and marionette folds
 Submalar concavities
 Recession of chin with deepening mental crease
 Prejowl sulcus and jowl formation
 Preauricular hollowing
Overall facial shape
 Proportions fall off from the ideal

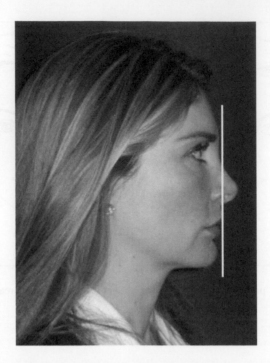

Figure 7.3 The "ideal" profile demonstrating alignment of the base of the glabella, subnasale, and chin with a vertical line drawn perpendicular to the Frankfort plane. This profile line enables one to easily assess recession of the chin.

examined for fullness. For the lower third of the face, assess the perioral region for furrows and concavities beyond the nasolabial and marionette folds. The subnasale will tend to sink as volume around the nose is lost, causing the nasal tip to droop. The corners of the mouth should be supported by volume. The profile should reveal the chin in alignment with the subnasale and glabella with the head held in a Frankfort horizontal plane (a standardized horizontal plane based on a line drawn through the superior aspect of the external auditory canal and infraorbital plane) (Fig. 7.3). The mandibular border should be smooth from chin to mandibular angle, without interruption from a prejowl defect or jowl protruberance. The submalar area should have some contour and tapering but no concavities. The preauricular area is another area to assess for flattening or hollowing.

The third assessment is to determine the areas where volume should be added in order to enhance the patient's overall beauty. To aid in this part of the examination, the patient should bring a favorite photograph taken 5 to 10 years earlier for comparison to a recent photograph. Specific areas that enhance beauty are the arch and contour of the brow, the fullness and apex of the malar mound, and the fullness and balance of the lips. Enhancement of

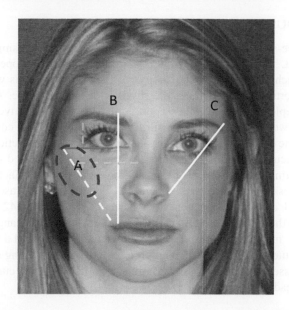

Figure 7.4 Guidelines for optimal cheek, lip, and brow aesthetics. *Dotted white line* should bisect an angled cheek oval (*dotted red line*), which extends as high as the lash line. The "A" represents the apex of the cheek at the intersection of a horizontal line approximately two-thirds down the nose and a vertical line midway between the brow and lateral canthus. Line B shows the ideal lip width from the medial limbus to the commissure. Line C represents brow length from the ala to the lateral canthus to the lateral brow. The apex of the brow should be above the lateral limbus or above the lateral canthus.

these areas will vary according to the patient's ethnicity, individual preference, current style, and facial structure, although some general guidelines exist, which may help with the analysis. The aesthetics of the arch of the brow have been described as maximizing the height at the lateral limbus of the eye and extending the length of the brow to intersect with a line drawn from the ala through the lateral canthus of the eye (Fig. 7.4) (34). The ideal location of the malar apex has been analyzed by many (35–40). One quick guideline is that the apex of the malar cheek should be at the intersection of a vertical line drawn between the brow and the lateral canthus and a horizontal line two-thirds down the nose (Fig. 7.4). Beautiful lips should be full, yet natural with four distinct "pillows" of volume: two of the upper and two of the lower lips, their width should fall between the medial limbus of the eyes, and the height of the upper lip should be 10% to 25% less than that of the lower one (Fig. 7.4) (41). The aesthetics of the brow, cheek, and lips should certainly be discussed with the patient so that individual preferences are expressed. It impresses upon the patient that the physician is interested not only in restoring facial volume but also in enhancing beauty.

AUTOLOGOUS FAT TRANSFER

AFT is a three-step procedure consisting of harvesting, processing, and transferring the fat. A review of the literature reveals that the proper method of performing each step has been the subject of debate. An issue is which factors are most important in determining the survival of the adipocyte. Although the literature is replete with anecdotal reports, there are few objective studies and definitive answers are lacking. The difficulty in establishing consensus is a reflection of the difficulty in measuring outcome. There is no practical method to objectively document results other than photography. Transferred fat cannot be labeled or distinguished from recipient site fat cells with a distinct histological marker. Successive imaging with magnetic resonance or ultrasonography is expensive and exposes the patient to unnecessary radiation (42). Measuring outcome is further complicated by variable rates of aging and changes in weight over time. We must, therefore, rely on photographic results until a better means of assessing outcome is available. New three-dimensional imaging systems hold promise for assessing fat survival over time, but their expense currently limits their widespread use (43).

Harvesting

Donor Site

The optimal donor site has not been unequivocally established. Many choose the outer thigh as the ideal site because of its nonfibrous nature and relative avascularity. The rationale is that the least vascularized tissue will best survive the initial hypoxic period after transfer. Two studies support that concept. Hudson et al. found that adipocytes from the buttock and outer thigh areas are the largest and have the greatest lipogenic activity (44). Ullman et al. injected fat from various sites into nude mice and found the outer thigh fat to have the lowest resorption rate (45). However, many patients desiring improvement of a gaunt facial appearance have very little body fat and one must obtain fat wherever possible. Areas that are diet-resistant, such as the knee, are often recommended in that, at least theoretically, the transplanted cells will be stable whether the patient gains or loses weight over time. An opposing study by Rohrich et al. found no difference among four different body sites (thigh, flank, knee, abdomen) by measuring adipocyte viability in vitro with colorimetric assays (46).

Use of Lidocaine

Some studies indicate that lidocaine has a negative effect on fat cell viability, whether its concentration is 1.0% or diluted to 0.1% (47,48). The effect could be removed by rinsing with saline. In contrast to these earlier studies, Keck et al. examined the effect of various local anesthetic solutions on the viability of preadipocytes in vitro and found the opposite to be true (49). After incubation for 30 minutes, simulating the time of clinical exposure, cell viability was found to be highest with lidocaine 1% at over 80% viability versus articaine at 55% and prilocaine at 26%. Of interest, when the articaine was diluted tenfold, the viability increased to 85%. This study of preadipocytes may help to explain why lidocaine has been used for decades with apparent success for donor site anesthesia. Differing dilutions of tumescent anesthesia have been recommended for donor site anesthesia with or without epinephrine. Amar recommends infiltrating Klein's solution much like a ring block around the core of fat to be harvested in order to minimize contact with lidocaine. Others recommend the use of Ringer's lactate rather than normal saline, reasoning that glucose-containing solution may enhance fat cell viability (50).

Harvesting Technique

Utilizing an enzymatic assay of fat cell damage, Lalikos et al. showed that harvesting by suction versus direct excision of fat did not increase apparent damage to the fat cell (51). Other studies have also demonstrated that fat cells harvested by syringe, machine aspiration, or direct excision all appear to have similar viability. Suction aspiration at low-level negative pressure did not appear to rupture cells in two studies, although partial breakage was seen at negative pressures of 700 mmHg and higher (52,53).

Syringe aspiration with low-level negative pressures is most often recommended. Those advocating the gentlest handling suggest 10-mLsyringes to minimize vacuum pressures with the plunger held back no more than 2 to 3 mL (Fig. 7.5) (22,50). Other experienced surgeons report harvesting with larger 20 to 60-mL syringes without apparent harm to the adipocytes, as documented with cell culture for up to two months (54). Although various cannulae and needles have been recommended, Shiffman and Mirrafati compared harvesting and reinjection with 2.5- to 3.0-mm cannulae and an 18-gauge needle. None of these caused disruption of fat cells histologically (55). However, needles smaller than 18 gauge did disrupt adipocyte histologically.

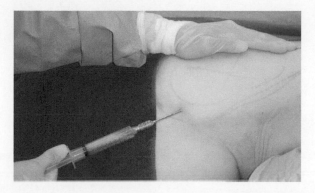

Figure 7.5 Gentle harvesting with a Klein 12-gauge Finesse™ cannula and a 10-mL syringe held back with 1 to 2 mL of pressure.

PROCESSING THE FAT

The next issue after harvesting the fat is whether or not it requires further processing before injection. Experts agree on the first step, which is to stand the syringes upright for a period of 15 to 60 minutes to allow separation into supranatant and infranatant fractions. The infranatant fluid is then drained off the bottom and the oil fraction on top is decanted off. In a survey of experienced cosmetic surgeons, 62% washed the fat with saline or Ringer's lactate to remove lidocaine or blood (56). Blood is thought by some to stimulate phagocytosis of fat cells (57). In Sommer's review, all authors in the referenced studies agreed that blood in transplanted fat accelerates its degradation (26).

Rather than rinse, many surgeons prefer to centrifuge the fat. A recent survey of 508 plastic surgeons revealed that 47% centrifuge fat, 29% rinse fat, and 12% transfer the fat directly without any processing (58). Centrifugation has been shown to separate fat cells from blood products, proteases, free lipids, and lipases that may degrade freshly grafted adipocytes (59). Various speeds and time intervals for centrifugation have been recommended. Histologically, fat cells centrifuged for 10 to 60 seconds at 3600 rpm show no evidence of cell damage, although cells centrifuged for 15 minutes have been shown to have distorted morphology (52,55).

Whether or not centrifugation removes lidocaine has not been demonstrated. Centrifugation does concentrate fat cells resulting in a larger number of cells per milliliter of volume transferred and a more cohesive strand of fat (Fig. 7.6). When 10 mL of fat is centrifuged at 3600 rpm for three minutes, there is a volume loss of approximately 30% to 40% of additional infranatant fluid (Fig. 7.7). In one of the few controlled studies, a double-blind comparison of fat

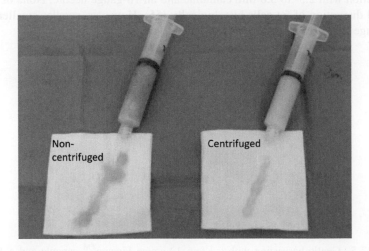

Figure 7.6 Centrifuged fat consisting of a more concentrated, more cohesive strand of fat than noncentrifuged fat.

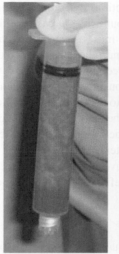
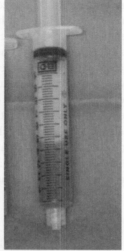

Upright x 1 hour   Centrifuged x 3 minutes

Figure 7.7 On the left, separation of infranatant and supranatant fat after one hour of sitting upright. On the right, after centrifugation at 3600 rpm for three minutes, the fat is compacted and additional infranatant fluid is separated.

transfer to the dorsum of the hands with centrifuged versus noncentrifuged fat the centrifuged hand was found to have improved longevity and aesthetic results at the three- and five-month follow-up visits in 100% of patients (Fig. 7.8) (60). The author now routinely utilizes centrifuged fat in essentially all cases. Some

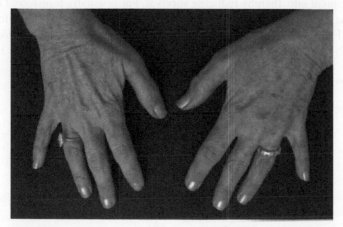

Centrifuged, 3 years later

Figure 7.8 Before and three years after AFT to dorsum of hands. Note better longevity on patient's left with centrifuged versus noncentrifuged fat on right.

advocate centrifuged fat for facial correction, but noncentrifuged fat for larger volume transfers into breasts, biceps, or buttocks—areas in which lumpiness has been noted with centrifuged fat (50). One must use sterilized canisters or sleeves within the centrifuge, as *Pseudomonas* and other pathogens have been cultured from centrifuges (61). New devices, recently approved by the FDA, enable suction of adipocytes followed by suction of excess fluids in a closed system (62,63). Clinical experience is needed to assess the utility of these devices. Recently, Moscatello et al. examined the addition of collagenase during fat processing with the goal of dissociating the fat graft into smaller cellular packets (64). In vitro ceiling culture showed greater than 80% viability compared to less than 50% for nondigested fat. Others have recommended the addition of glycogen or growth factors, but definite benefit has yet to be demonstrated (65,66).

Transfer Techniques

There are various AFT techniques that have been proposed over the years; its usual placement is within the subcutaneous fat (24,67,68). The suggested degree of overcorrection has decreased through the years, and now minimal or no overcorrection is recommended (23,24,50). Not only is fat survival improved with small volumes of fat, but downtime is also minimized. As a general rule, postoperative edema is proportional to the amount transferred (69,70). Retrograde injection through a 14- to 25-gauge needle or, more commonly, a blunt-tipped cannula is usually suggested. Shiffman's study demonstrated that needles smaller than 18 gauge caused damage to adipocytes (71). Another reason to favor blunt-tipped cannulae is the reduced risks of bleeding and intravascular injection. Those who favor needles argue that cannulae pass through tissue with more friction and trauma, which may cause increased bleeding and inflammation in the recipient site, thereby reducing survival. Fat is usually transferred from the harvesting syringe to smaller syringes for injection with a female-to-female adaptor (Fig. 7.9). Various-sized syringes are recommended ranging from 1-ml (22,59,72) to 3-ml (68) to 10-ml (55,70) syringe. The author prefers the 1-ml

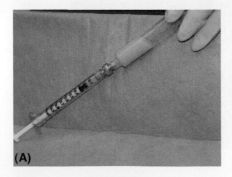
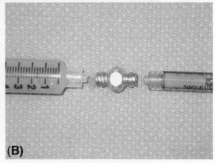

Figure 7.9   Fat transferred to 1-mL syringes (**A**) via a female-to-female transfer hub (**B**).

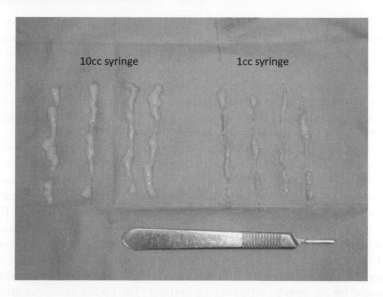

Figure 7.10 Retrograde strands of fat are thinner in diameter when passed through a 1-ml syringe on right versus a 10-ml syringe on left.

syringe, as less pressure is required to empty it and thinner diameter fat strands are produced (Fig. 7.10). Fat is then injected as the cannula is withdrawn and small strands of fat are placed.

Other techniques for AFT involve placement of fat in multiple tissue planes. Coleman coined the phrase "Lipostructure" to describe his intricate layering of minute parcels of fat throughout multiple tissue planes, not only in the subcutaneous plane but also adjacent to bone, fascia, and muscle (22). Each droplet of fat is placed "within 1.5 mm of living vascularized tissue". Typically, 30 or 40 passes are required to empty a 1-mL syringe with a blunt-tipped 17-gauge or 18-gauge cannula. Quantities injected for a full face often exceed 100 mL. Because the fat is viewed as a living graft, it is handled gently with atraumatic harvesting, no rinsing, and brief centrifugation for 30 seconds. Coleman reports long-term results with his method in the order of years. Before and after photographs suggest that Lipostructure may replace the need for rhytidectomy. The single most significant drawback to this method is the marked edema seen for weeks or months postoperatively because of the large volumes placed. The benefit of dramatic panfacial correction must be weighed against the extended recovery period for the patient.

To circumvent prolonged edema for the patient, Donofrio modified Coleman's procedure with a method of "facial rebalancing," also involving the entire face but with repeated smaller procedures (6–12 procedures) over a one- to two-year period (59). Fresh fat is utilized the first time, but in most patients frozen fat is injected on subsequent visits. The entire face is treated with smaller total quantities (approximately 20–30 mL), which reduces the downtime for patients to 1 to 10 days depending on the extent of the procedure. Fat is processed atraumatically and injected with blunt-tipped cannulae with the intricate, repetitive-pass, layered method first developed by Coleman. Donofrio not only focuses on replacing fat but also addresses areas of fat hypertrophy that are found in the aging face. Microliposuction of the jowls and other areas is typically performed during the fat transfer procedure for aesthetic rebalancing.

The author prefers a third technique called FAMI or fat autograft muscle injection since its introduction to the United States in 2001 (73). Most cosmetic surgeons agree that an abundantly vascularized recipient site for transplanted fat will result in optimal survival of the fat, an opinion confirmed by several histological studies (25,55,56,74). French anatomist and plastic surgeon, Roger Amar, has incorporated this principle into a technique in which fat is injected into or immediately adjacent to the muscles of facial expression. The concept of FAMI was inspired by a study in 1996 by Guerrerosantos, in which he demonstrated five-year survival of fat in rat muscle (75). Muscle thickness continued to increase for six months following fat grafting. The FAMI technique involves full-face volume correction following the template of the patient's anatomy, namely the origin and insertion of various muscle groups. Volumes placed range from approximately 20 mL to 100 mL or more utilizing a set of blunt-tipped cannulae, which are curved and angled to conform to the contours of the face and underlying skeletal features (Fig. 7.11). There is more efficiency and less apparent trauma than methods by Coleman and Donofrio, who describe over

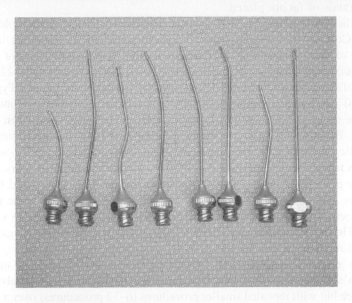

Figure 7.11 FAMI injection cannulae.

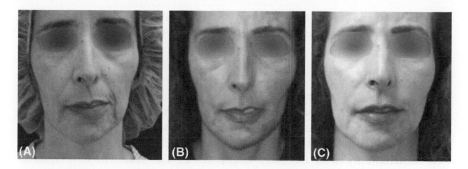

Figure 7.12 (A) 48-year-old patient with traumatic injury to left side of the face, postsurgical correction of bone, before FAMI. (B) Six months and (C) 12 months after corrective FAMI. Three sessions of 19.8, 10, and 11 ml were performed.

30 rapid, repetitive passes to empty a single syringe. With FAMI, a 1-mL syringe is emptied in one to three passes. The fat is placed along vectors that parallel blood supply, minimizing trauma to the vessels. Patients are able to return to work in three to seven days depending on volumes placed. Amar has reported longevity of three to five years with this method (30). The technique has evolved over time, and Amar now also utilizes supraperiosteal injections of highly centrifuged fat containing a high concentration of adipose-derived stem cells. In vitro, these cells have the potential to differentiate into adipocytes, bone, and other tissues (76).

FAMI can be performed as a full-face volume correction or for localized volume loss such as the lips, tear-trough deformity, chin, or perioral regions. It is ideal after rhytidectomy in patients with thin, overly taut skin. FAMI can be helpful in reconstructive surgery after injury or trauma (Fig. 7.12). It is also indicated in conjunction with liposuction of the neck for replacing volume of the chin, mandibular border, prejowl sulcus, and lower perioral regions (77). In restoring the muscle sling of the face and correcting for bone loss, the overlying skin redrapes in the smooth, uninterrupted contours of youth.

Preoperative Preparation

Whatever the technique, a preoperative history and physical examination are performed to screen for serious medical conditions, concomitant infections, bleeding diatheses, medications, and allergies. Medications containing aspirin and nonsteroidal anti-inflammatory agents are discontinued two weeks before surgery. Vitamin E and certain herbal formulations should be discontinued before surgery. Prophylactic oral antibiotic therapy is started the night before the procedure: cephalexin 500 mg orally twice daily for seven days or minocycline 100 mg orally once or twice daily for penicillin-allergic patients. To minimize potential bruising, mephyton may be prescribed or bromelain may be recommended (78). The choice for the donor site is discussed with patients in advance. Benefits and risks are reviewed, as well as the postoperative sequelae.

FAMI Procedure

Amar's harvesting and processing techniques include utilizing the medial knee as his preferred donor site, and processing of the fat with centrifugation at 3600 rpm for three minutes. Injection into the muscles is based on anatomic knowledge of the origin, insertion, and plane of each muscle to be injected as well as familiarity with the bony landmarks of the skull (79–81). Specific injection cannulae have been developed for various muscle groups, allowing for smooth passage of the cannula. The cannula is directed distally to the origin or insertion of the muscle and the fat is injected in a retrograde fashion with low injection pressure. An assistant records the quantities placed along the muscles on each side to assure symmetry or, if necessary, to record correction of pre-existing asymmetry. There are three ways the surgeon determines that he or she is injecting in the muscle. For certain muscles, such as the depressor anguli oris, the bundle palpably enlarges as the enveloping fascia is filled. Other muscles, like the zygomaticus minor, are very thin, not palpable, and the surgeon must rely on bony anatomic landmarks to inject as close as possible to the muscle. With other muscle groups, a loss of resistance is the clue that the cannula has penetrated the fascia and is within the muscle. After injections along the muscle, additional injections are often performed directly in the subcutaneous layer or deeper at the supraperiosteal level. Anesthesia for this procedure is achieved with nerve blocks supplemented with oral or intravenous sedation depending on individual patient sensitivity.

A typical FAMI injection for the full face starts cephalad to caudad (Table 7.3). The glabellar muscles are injected followed by the frontalis. Fat is then placed under the brow, with the non-dominant hand lifting up the soft tissue

Table 7.3 FAMI Treatment Protocol

Sterile prep and drape
Donor site anesthesia with Klein's tumescent formula
Nerve blocks of the face
Gentle harvesting with 10-mL syringe
Syringes held upright and intranatant fluid discarded
Full 10-ml syringe centrifuged at 3600 rpm for three minutes
Oil and infranatant fractions discarded
Transfer to 1-ml syringes
Inject cephalad to caudad each muscle group, bilaterally
Inject supraperiosteal and subcutaneous areas as indicated
Postoperative checks at 24 hours and one week
Evaluate for touch-up session at 6- to 12-month intervals
Touch-up injections with <10 ml of frozen fat

Table 7.4 Muscles of the Cheeks

Muscle	Plane	Cannula #
Zygomaticus minor	Superficial	4
Levator labii superioris aleque nasi	Mid	1
Levator labii superioris	Mid	5
Levator anguli oris	Deep	7
Zygomaticus major	Mid	10

of the brow, allowing the injection of the fat to be sandwiched between fibers of the obicularis oculi. The fossa temporalis is then injected in a subcutaneous plane because the muscle is less accessible in this region. The cheek involves injection of multiple muscles per the order given in Table 7.4. One of the most dramatic injections is along the zygomaticus minor because the injection begins at the muscle's origin on the zygoma and extends over the cheek and then under and medial to the nasolabial fold. As fat is injected, the base of the nose is lifted and the cheek–lip junction becomes a smooth continuous contour (Fig. 7.13).

The perioral region is the key region of the lower face. There are three deep injections here; of these, two are not on the muscle but are supraperiosteal and are used to fill up the upper and lower sulci below the teeth, which deepen with age because of boney changes. Injections of small quantities along the sulci help to support the lips and lift the overlying soft tissue (Fig. 7.14). The muscles that are potentially injected are listed in Table 7.5, along with the numbered cannula utilized in that region of the face. Intraoperatively, the quantities injected in each muscle are recorded. In addition to muscle and supraperiosteal injections, fat may be placed in the subcutaneous plane to add symmetry and beauty, especially in the malar area and lips. Atrophic fat compartments of the face may need additional filling. For example, the lateral compartment of the

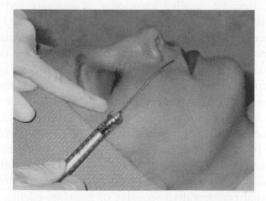

Figure 7.13 Injection of the zygomaticus minor with cannula 4, crossing the nasolabial fold.

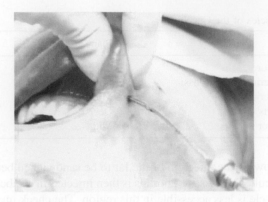

Figure 7.14 Supraperiosteal injection of right alveolar sulcus with cannula 5. Filling deeply along the bone will lift concavities of chin and marionette areas.

Table 7.5 Muscles of the Lower Face

Muscles	Plane	Cannulae
Levator muscles (see Table 7.4)	Mid-deep	1, 5, 7
Depressor labii inferioris	Mid	7
Depressor anguli oris	Mid	5
Mentalis	Deep	1
Buccinator	Deep	5
Risorius	Mid	3
Platysma	Mid	3
Obicularis oris	Mid	10

face is often more atrophic after rhytidectomy than other fat compartments. This manifests as preauricular hollowing and is best corrected by filling in the subcutaneous plane. Because detailed knowledge of anatomy and facial aging is essential for performing the FAMI technique, it is best learned through a live workshop or preceptorship with an experienced cosmetic surgeon.

The postoperative course of FAMI is uneventful. There is essentially no pain. Mild-to-moderate purpura is common, although it may not appear until some of the edema subsides on the second or third day. Edema is the most significant symptom and patients need to be warned in advance or they will be concerned that too much fat has been placed. The recovery period will depend on the quantities placed. With a full-face correction of 70 mL or more, the patient may require 7 to 10 days of downtime. In a preliminary report, the author utilized smaller total volumes, 20 to 30 mL on average, which reduced the downtime to three to five days (82). Complications of this technique have not been reported except for the usual postoperative sequelae of bruising, edema, and temporary palpable lumpiness, which is generally not visible. Symmetry and consistent, predictable results are reasons FAMI is the author's preferred AFT method (83).

Table 7.6 Complications of AFT

Expected: edema, purpura
Overcorrection
Fat hyperatrophy with weight gain
Fat necrosis
Cysts/calcification
Infection
Vascular occlusion
Muscle injury

Complications of AFT

The complication rate is low and rarely significant with all AFT techniques (Table 7.6). Overcorrection is probably the most common complication, particularly in the infraorbital area. Visible, superficial nodules may develop with overcorrection of this area or from injecting too large a parcel of fat too superficially (72). Caution is advised in this area if it is to be injected at all. Experienced surgeons recommend that very minute quantities are injected in the periorbital area with each pass of a 1-mL syringe (72,84). Limiting the quantity to 0.5 ml per eye has eliminated this complication in the author's practice. Overcorrection may be difficult to treat, but low-dose intralesional steroid injection, repeated massage, ultrasound, and excision have been suggested.

Other potential complications sometimes seen after AFT include fat hypertrophy, particularly following weight gain after fat augmentation, which may require surgical revision (85). The precision and symmetry of the FAMI technique appears to mitigate this problem so that the face is still balanced regardless of changes in weight. Fat necrosis may occur on occasion resulting in extrusion of fat, and cysts or calcifications (86,87). Infection is another potential complication, with reports of infection with *staphylococcus*, *streptococcus*, and mycobacteria (68,72,88). Patients need to be screened adequately for concomitant, recurrent, or chronic infections, particularly of adjacent facial areas such as sinus, dental, or ocular regions (88). These infections must be adequately treated before the procedure. The use of prophylactic antibiotics is generally recommended in all patients. In addition, AFT should be carried out as a sterile procedure. Because the centrifuge has been the source of infection with *pseudomonas*, sterile centrifuge sleeves should be utilized (61).

The most serious potential complication of fat augmentation is vascular occlusion caused by the release of emboli from inadvertent intravascular injection. Blindness has been reported following fat injections of the glabellar lines (89), and also from injection of the nasolabial fold (90,91). Middle cerebral artery occlusion and ocular fat embolism have also been reported following fat injection of the face (92,93). Yoon and co-workers reported an acute fatal stroke immediately following AFT (94). Reports have implicated sharp instrumentation and/or high injection pressures with 10-mL syringes. Use of blunt-tipped cannulae and initial withdrawal of the plunger will minimize the risk of vascular penetration and intravascular injection. Retrograde filler placement, 1-mL syringes, and low injection pressures further reduce the risk of intravascular injection. When dramatic blanching of the skin—indicating vascular compromise—occurs, Wexler advises placing the patient in Trendelenberg position, applying nitroglycerin paste, and massaging the area until the flush of the skin returns (95). With intramuscular injection of autologous fat, another potential complication is dysfunction of facial muscles. Although not reported by Amar, weakness of facial muscles of mastication has been observed when fat is injected in the muscles (96). For that reason, the masseter muscle is not injected per the FAMI procedure. As well, the curved and angled cannulae used for FAMI glide smoothly along the muscle's trajectory and minimize injury.

Longevity of Results

The biggest dilemma in fat augmentation is predicting what percentage of fat will "take" and how long the results will last. The literature contains few objective studies regarding the longevity of transplanted fat. Horl et al. demonstrated a 49% volume loss at 3 months, 55% loss at 6 months, and negligible loss between 9 and 12 months utilizing magnetic resonance imaging of fat transplants (97). Ultrasound imaging has been utilized to demonstrate long-term correction up to one year in patients with defects because of various disease processes (98,99). Another prospective study evaluated longevity using CT scanning with three-dimensional volume analysis in HIV-positive patients treated with the Coleman method. Not only did fat endure at one year, but also—for unknown reasons—there was a tendency for the volume to increase from the second to twelfth month (100). Sadick and Hudgins used a marker of fatty acid composition that was specific to the donor site (101). He was able to demonstrate a one-year persistence of that marker in the recipient site in one of the six patients. In the other five, the donor site marker was undetectable. He speculated that recipient site factors may have caused conversion of the donor site marker to the fatty acid composition of the recipient site.

Animal studies have shown long-term survival of autologous fat. Nguyen and coworkers found persistence of transplanted fat in rats at nine months only when fat was injected into the muscle (102). Fat injected into the subcutaneous plane was completely absorbed. Guerrerosantos reported five-year survival of fat when injected into rat muscle (75).

Studies in which results were based on photographic images or physician assessments have reported long-term results varying from "disappointing" to many years (2,18,50,68,70). Some have noted the longest survival when the recipient site is relatively immobile, such as the fixed scars of linear morphea (23), the forehead (67), the infraorbital area (50), or the back of the hands (103,104). In a study of scleroderma-induced facial scars, these results were

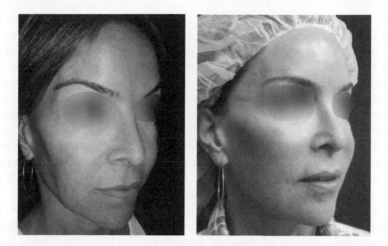

Figure 7.15 Long-term survival four years after procedure. Patient had touch-up with frozen fat twice, each with 10 ml. Present photo is one year after last touch-up.

corroborated: the forehead had the greatest retention of 51% to 75% at one year, while scars of the chin and nose showed poor correction of less than 25% (105). The most mobile area of the face—the lips—has been least responsive to long-term correction in other reports (50,106). Eremia and Newman found that longevity was related to recipient site (106). Good-to-excellent results were seen at five to eight months for the nasolabial and melolabial folds and poor results were observed in the lip and glabella. Perez notes more permanent results in younger patients (107). Based on the limited objective data, animal studies, and empirical and sometimes conflicting reports from experienced cosmetic surgeons, one can conclude that long-term fat survival is achievable. Per the author's clinical experience with FAMI, this duration is from a few to many years (Fig. 7.15). Further studies are ongoing to define the factors resulting in optimal survival.

USE OF FROZEN FAT

To avoid a sterile reharvesting procedure, many experienced fat injectors freeze harvested fat for later touch-up procedures and report satisfactory results (59,70,108,109). In the author's practice, harvested fat is stored in an industrial freezer for up to three years. The freezer needs to be in compliance with individual state's guidelines and in some states be registered yearly as a tissue bank. Many patients choose to have additional procedures, particularly in the perioral area where the survival of the fat seems to be relatively poor, most likely because of constant movement of the newly grafted tissue. A frozen-fat session typically utilizes 10 ml or less and is used in particular situations, including patients with weight loss after the initial procedure, cautious patients who initially wanted to be very conservative and want more at a later time, or, most commonly, patients trying to offset the ongoing aging process by adding volume every one to two years. A typical protocol in the author's practice is to have one larger session of FAMI with 30 to 40 mL of fresh fat, expecting downtime of five to seven days. This is followed by one to three touch-up sessions, at intervals of 6 to 12 months with 10 mL of frozen fat. These smaller sessions are relatively quick office visits and heal over the weekend. Variations from this protocol include injection sessions monthly or every other month for one to two years with frozen fat for gradual sequential augmentation (59). Coleman prefers to repeat the entire initial session every few years as needed with fresh fat. Fournier advocates periodic injections every few years to keep pace with the aging process (108). He also regularly uses frozen fat as needed for touch-up procedures.

A few studies have addressed the issue of the viability of frozen fat. Histological studies by Takasu and Takasu have demonstrated that frozen and thawed adipocytes are identical to those of normal tissue (110). They have further reported long-term retention of fat that had been frozen for up to seven years. Shoshani et al. compared frozen fat versus fresh fat injected into nude mice (111). Assessments by clinical observation, weight and volume measurement, and histological parameters demonstrated successful take at 15 weeks in both groups with no statistically significant difference in volume at 15 weeks. In a side-by-side comparison study of fresh versus frozen fat injected to the dorsum of the hands, it was found that frozen fat lasted at least as long and sometimes longer at three-month and five-month intervals (112). Aesthetically, the hand treated with the frozen fat was preferred at the three-month and five-month follow-up and patients noted less postoperative edema of the hand, a finding corroborated by Saylan (109). Another study compared the viability of adipocytes frozen with either of the four methods: snap frozen in liquid nitrogen without media, frozen at $-20°C$ without media, incubated at $37°C$ with 10% bovine serum, or incubated without media. The fat frozen at $-20°C$ showed only a slight drop in mitochondrial activity at eight days, whereas all other methods had a more than 60% drop in mitochondrial activity (113). However, other studies reject the use of frozen fat. Lawrence found no viable adipocytes in frozen aspirates measured by cell culture (114). Research regarding the viability of frozen fat is ongoing with some exploring the role of cryopreservatives (115,116). Newer studies indicate that preadipocytes may survive the freezing process (117).

VOLUMIZING WITH SYNTHETIC AGENTS

Facial volumizing with material other than autologous fat has been a challenge because of the sheer quantity of product required and the cost of these fillers. In the relatively recent past, only bovine collagen was available in the United States. The short duration and relatively thin consistency of these products meant that numerous syringes would be necessary for a fleeting result. Volumizing with bovine collagen was simply economically prohibitive for the majority of patients. New, more robust products with longer duration are now available, thereby bypassing the harvesting portion of AFT and the need for a sterile procedure. In a relatively quick office visit, the patient can have a fuller, more youthful face, often with a more predictable duration than AFT. In addition, synthetic fillers make it possible to volumize a very thin patient with too little adipose tissue for harvesting. Contemporary injectable filling agents may be classified by material, duration, or mechanism of action (Table 7.1). The latter classification by mechanism refers to *replacement* fillers, which occupy space in the deep dermis or other layers, and *stimulatory* fillers, which replace volume in part by stimulating fibroblast activity with resultant collagen production.

Volumizing with synthetic fillers is typically performed with hyaluronic acid (HA), calcium hydroxylapatite (CaHA), poly-L-lactic acid (PLLA), or some combination of these fillers. Other fillers may be utilized, but some have recently exited the market (e.g., porcine collagen), whereas others are typically used only for deep lines (polymethyl methacrylate). As well, silicon is not FDA-approved as a cosmetic filling agent in the United States.

Hyaluronic acid is a natural component of the connective tissue matrix in which collagen and elastic fibers are embedded. HA is highly hydrophilic, which increases tissue hydration and enhances dermal volume. Synthetic HA gels are considered spacers, although they have been shown to have a minor biostimulatory effect as well because of stretching of the myofibroblast (118). The majority of HA products in the United States are derived from bacterial culture with the exception of Hylaform® derived from avian culture. The duration of HA products is 3 to 12 months depending on the concentration of HA, the extent of cross-linking of HA, and the location of injection. Skin testing is not required. The HAs have a soft-gel consistency and are useful for focal areas for facial restructuring, such as the tear trough, lateral brow, and mid-cheek defects (119). For volumizing, thicker HAs, such as Juvederm® Ultra Plus (Allergan, Irvine, California, U.S.) and Perlane® (Medicis Aesthetics, Scottsdale, Arizona, U.S.), provide more structure and possibly longer duration. A major benefit of these agents is reversibility with hyaluronidase should a problem arise (120).

Calcium hydroxylapatite is a major mineral component of bone that is suspended in an aqueous gel matrix, also containing glycerin and sodium hydroxycellulose (Radiesse®, BioForm Medical, San Mateo, California, U.S.). The gel is absorbed six to eight weeks after injection while the mineral microspheres persist and serve as a scaffold for concomitant biostimulatory effects on collagen production. The microspheres degrade into calcium and phosphate ions over time and the augmentation diminishes over a period reported to be two to five years, but in clinical practice is 12 to 18 months. Because of its high viscosity and to reduce the discomfort associated with the injection, the product is often mixed or "swished" with 0.15 to 0.5 ml or more of 1% lidocaine to enable smoother injection through 27- to 28-gauge needles. The author prefers a 1¼-in length for injecting retrograde threads of the material. CaHA is placed more deeply than HA, in the subdermal or supra-periosteal plane. The product is bulky and is useful for lifting and filling the malar cheek and filling deeper furrows such as the nasolabial fold and mari-onette lines. It has also been observed to require less volume to achieve correction than other fillers with one study demonstrating that it takes 30% less volume to fill nasolabial folds compared to an HA product (121,122). A syringe of Radiesse® contains 1.5 ml of product often enabling correction of several deep lines or both cheeks with one syringe. Radiesse is contraindicated in the lips because of the risk of submucosal nodules, with a reported inci-dence of up to 20% (123). Caution is advised in the tear trough area where the skin is thin and nodules from overcorrection or muscle movement are quite visible. Many injectors, including the author, avoid using this product in the tear trough altogether. Other experienced injectors dilute the product even more when injecting in this area (124).

Poly-L-lactic acid is the newest agent for facial volumizing, first approved by the FDA in 2004 for HIV-associated facial lipoatrophy and in 2009 for cos-metic use. PLLA microparticles are α-hydroxy acid polymers suspended in sodium carboxycellulose and mannitol (Sculptra®, Sanofi-Aventis US, Bridge-water, New Jersey, U.S.). The package insert recommends that the product be reconstituted with 3 to 5 ml of sterile water two hours before use. Clinical experience with PLLA has led to more dilute solutions in order to minimize the risk of subcutaneous nodules with this product. The author utilizes an 8-cc dilution, consisting of 1 ml of 1% lidocaine and 7 ml of sterile water. In our practice, PLLA is always mixed 24 hours ahead of time and agitated with a vortex mixer immediately before use to achieve a uniform suspension. The dilution, time of reconstitution before use, interval between treatments (one month or more), even distribution of product, and patient massage afterwards are key factors that minimize the risk of subcutaneous nodules with this product (125). Skin testing is not necessary. The product is placed in deeper planes, subdermal and supra-periosteal, but never superficial, and always with care to inject an even distri-bution (126). The implanted PLLA microparticles spread evenly along the tissue have been likened to "seeds" that then induce a local tissue reaction characterized by an increase in fibroblasts and new collagen production. The treatment must be staged in monthly and longer intervals and the result is a gradual one over many months. This is not a product for patients desiring immediate correction. How-ever, many patients appreciate the gradual improvement rather than looking corrected overnight. Patients also like the control to stop when they achieve their desired result, as many fear an overfilled appearance. Once achieved, the aug-mentation lasts 18 to 30 months according to reports.

FACIAL VOLUMIZING WITH SYNTHETIC FILLERS

The face is prepped with an antibacterial cleanser and the proposed treatment areas are marked using a surgical pen or a washable marker and confirmed with

Table 7.7   Volumizing with Synthetic Fillers

Key areas
  Temple
  Lateral brow
  Malar cheek and apex
  Nasojugal fold
  Mid-cheek crease
  Preauricular hollow
  Marionette folds/commissures
  Prejowl sulcus
  Mandibular border concavities

the patient. Because each syringe is costly, one must be more strategic with synthetic fillers by placement in key areas, so that the final result approximates full-face volumizing with AFT (Table 7.7). The procedure usually proceeds cephalad to caudad. Products are injected with a combination of techniques including retrograde linear threading, fanning, cross-fanning, and deep depot deposits (Figs 7.16–7.19).

The mid and upper forehead is rarely treated with synthetic volumizers as neurotoxins are usually the preferred treatment and the risks of intravascular injection and irregularities are greater. The exception is volumizing the temple and atrophic region immediately at and above the lateral brow to widen the narrowing aging face, restore the oval shape of the upper face, and give a modest brow lift. PLLA is the author's preferred agent for the temple because its watery nature enables withdrawal before injection to avoid intravascular injection and, when placed deeply under the temporal fascia, can be accomplished with one needle stick. The technique that is applicable in the temple is a deep depot injection, essentially burying a 5/8-in., 25-gauge needle, aspirating, and then injecting 1 ml of an 8-ml dilution. The temple is then filled in this deep plane. The product can also be directed laterally under the hairline if indicated. A second syringe can be directed above the lateral brow, placing approximately 0.2 to 0.5 mL and repeating with an additional 0.2 ml immediately under the brow by lifting up the orbicularis occuli muscle and placing a retrograde thread of 0.1 to 0.2 ml of product. HAs and CaHA can also be placed under the brow in a similar fashion in the supraperiosteal plane. The temples are not typically filled with these products because of the large quantities required and the inability to aspirate these products.

The malar region is one of the most satisfying regions to enhance, and any product can be utilized. Many strategies for the optimal malar cheek have been presented and debated in the literature. The model the author utilizes is modified from Swift's concept (127) shown in Figure 7.4. Products are generally placed deeply in the supraperiosteal region with a fanning and cross-fanning technique. If more lift is desired, more viscous agents, such as CaHA or thicker HAs, should

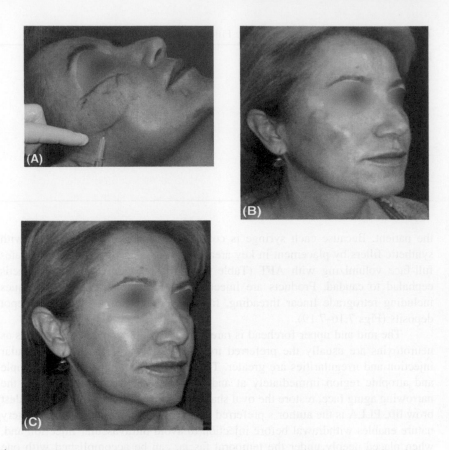

Figure 7.16 Lifting the cheek, NLF, marionette, and pre-jowl sulcus with calcium hydroxylapatite 1.5 ml for entire face. Treatment plan and bleb of local anesthesia shown in A. B—immediately after, C—one month follow up.

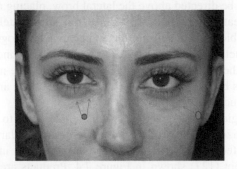

Figure 7.17 Treating the tear trough with HA. Gently flick the bone with the needle to ensure deep placement and place small aliquots along orbital rim.

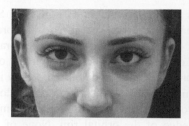
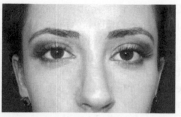

Figure 7.18 Before and three months after two sessions of HA, one month apart. First session used 0.15 ml on each side. Second session used 0.2 ml on each side.

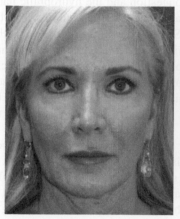
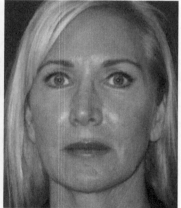

Figure 7.19 Before and one month after combination therapy with HA (1 ml to red portion of lips and 0.1 ml to each tear trough—0.1 ml per side) and 1 vial of PLLA to temples, medial and lateral cheek, and preauricular area. A neurotoxin was also placed in the glabella and lateral brow. Two vials of PLLA were placed at one month intervals over the previous three months for an overall total of three vials of PLLA.

be placed (Fig. 7.17). The apex of the oval of the malar cheek should be emphasized to enhance beauty and to catch the light reflex. This is done with either HA or CaHA by directing the needle under and deep to the apex and aiming upward to the immediate subdermal region and placing a small bolus of product for an immediate lift. PLLA in the malar cheek is placed in three levels: supraperiosteal, mid-subcutaneous plane, and, with small quantities, immediately subdermal. It is more difficult to create an apex with this product because of the risk of nodularity if too much is placed in a small focal area.

The anteromedial cheek and nasojugal fold are important to address as atrophy in this area results in a tired appearance. There is often a mid-cheek crease extending from the tear trough that should also be addressed. Any of the three types of filling agents can be placed here, although the author does not place CaHA in this region and prefers a medium-weight HA instead. Small quantities are recommended in a supraperiosteal plane. The infraorbital foramen should be palpated to avoid inadvertent injection of product into the foramen. While in this region, the needle can be directed up to the inferior edge of the infraorbital rim. Very small aliquots of product can then be placed deeply in the supraperiosteal plane with a depot or mini-thread under the tear trough following the contour of the bone (Fig. 7.17). The orbit is protected with the nondominant index finger placed along the superior edge of the orbital rim. None of these products is placed above the orbital rim to avoid nodularity and to minimize the risk of Tyndall effect. The emphasis is on small quantities in this region, such as 0.1 to 0.4 per side. Placement of 2 to 3 mL of HA has been associated with persistent edema because of lymphatic congestion and the hydrophilic nature of this material (128). It should be noted that patients are particularly disturbed by adverse effects in the infraorbital region. Some patients swell more than others in this region and a cautious approach is advised, particularly the first time this area is treated. Patients should be advised of potential adverse effects, including undercorrection, which is a reasonable approach in this area, with subsequent follow-up two to four weeks later for additional enhancement (Fig. 7.18). Use of reversible HA products is recommended, particularly the first time a tear trough is treated.

The lateral cheek and preauricular area are an excellent area for volumization and the author's product of choice is PLLA. This product is optimal for the broad, flat preauricular region from the subzygomatic area to the lateral mandibular border and angle. One to 2 ml of an 8-ml dilution are cross fanned with a 1½-in., 25-gauge needle in the mid to high subcuticular plane. Volumizing in this region replaces the atrophic lateral fat pad described by Rohrich and Pessa (9) and serves to pull back and lessen the appearance of the jowl (Fig. 7.19). Patients having undergone rhytidectomy in the past may be fibrotic in this area because of scarring from the procedure. PLLA should be placed under, not in, this fibrotic tissue. Other products, HA and CaHA, are not as useful for this broad, flat plane because they do not spread and may look uneven. If utilized in this area, diluting HA or CaHA with 0.2 to 0.5 ml of 1% lidocaine is helpful for a smoother flow and more even results.

Volumization of the lower face may be accomplished with any of the previously mentioned agents. In general, the more viscous fillers or repeated PLLA injections are needed for deeper chin defects or for chin enhancement, whereas the HAs are used for the lips and commissures. PLLA and CaHA are contraindicated in the lips because of the risk of nodularity. For deep marionette lines, the mental crease, and chin enhancement, a multilevel approach is taken, starting with deep retrograde threads of product fanned under the depressor muscles of the lip and the mentalis. Mid and high subcutaneous planes are filled again with a retrograde threading technique. In areas of maximum multidirectional muscle movement, all products have a risk of nodularity. For this reason, smaller quantities of CaHA or PLLA are placed in the commissure area.

Additional enhancement can then be achieved with the more forgiving HAs. Neurotoxins can be added to reduce movement and to extend the longevity of the filler.

Attention should also be given to disguising the jowl by creating a smooth mandibular border. Thicker HAs, CaHA, or PLLA are delivered similarly in retrograde linear threads in the prejowl sulcus medial to the jowl and also lateral to the jowl up to the mandibular angle, deep in the supraperiosteal plane. The entire sweep of a smooth, uninterrupted mandible creates a youthful appearance. The buccal and submalar areas may need to be addressed in some patients after all other areas are treated. This area is often tented and may be improved by filling superior and inferior to it. It is important not to overfill this area in order to maintain attractive tapering of the face; too much filler can weigh down the skin and inadvertently accentuate the jowl or give the face a rectangular shape. Small quantities are therefore placed in this region, preferably with lightweight HAs, PLLA, or diluted CaHA.

When volumizing with synthetic fillers, combination therapy and layering are often utilized, as one product may not be optimal in all areas (Fig. 7.19). Immediate massage is a component of treatment to assure smoothness. For PLLA, postoperative massage by the patient—25 times over a period of 5 to 10 days—is advised. With new patients and new injectors, focal areas can be performed initially, with more product added in subsequent visits, after gaining confidence with positive experience. Novice injectors should attend live workshops or receive adequate training with different products and preceptors. Anesthesia will vary according to the patient's tolerance, but injecting in the subcutaneous planes is surprisingly painless compared to dermal injections. Topical anesthetics may be adequate, particularly when the injectables are combined with lidocaine. The author often injects three to five blebs of local anesthetic per side, "numbing dots" at key injection points of the face in the first few minutes. The patient can then relax because the remainder of the session is essentially painless. Complications of synthetic filling agents are rarely serious but not uncommon, with bruising and swelling being the most frequent adverse effects. Nodules may occur, typically from excessive or too superficial product placement, but may improve spontaneously over two to three weeks. As opposed to the previously used bovine collagen, allergic reactions to modern synthetic filler agents are extremely rare.

CONCLUSION

Facial volumizing may be successfully performed with either autologous fat or synthetic fillers. With careful technique and attention to aesthetic details, volumizing is a low-risk and high-reward procedure. Increasing knowledge of facial aging has helped to target key areas for optimal rejuvenation so that, compared to AFT, reduced quantities of synthetic fillers are often sufficient. Given the plethora of available fillers with more to come in the future, it seems AFT could go the way of the dinosaur. There are several factors, however, that would seem to preclude this possibility. The first is the autologous nature of fat. There is no risk of long-term granulomas or immune effects, which will always appeal to patients. Second, fat has the potential for predictable, long-term survival unlike most synthetic fillers. New advances with fat processing and adipocyte stem cells hold promise for improved longevity, predictability, and results (129). Additionally, although much can be accomplished with synthetic fillers, the sheer volume of 50 to 100 ml that is often required for facial volume restoration renders synthetic fillers unaffordable for many patients. Finally, AFT is a creative, gratifying surgical procedure performed only by physicians and is therefore restricted from the realm of nonphysician providers and medical spas. For cosmetic surgeons and patients, the options continue to increase and the techniques and results continue to improve. Today's increasing "trend" in facial volumizing is sure to endure for decades to come.

REFERENCES

1. The American Society of Plastic Surgery 2006 and 2008 Procedure Statistics. Available at: http://www.plasticsurgery.org. Accessed January 2010.
2. Fournier PF. Syringe fat grafting. In: Narins RS, ed. Safe Liposuction and Fat Transfer. New York: Maral Dekkor, 2003:425–454.
3. Kahn DM, Shaw RB. Aging of the bony orbit: a three dimensional computed tomographic study. Aesthet Surg J 2008; 28(3):258–264.
4. Pessa J. An algorithm of facial aging. Verification of Lambros' theory by three-dimensional stereolithography, with reference to the pathogenesis of mid facial aging, scleral show, and the lateral suborbital trough deformity. Plast Reconstr Surg 2000; 106:479–488.
5. Pessa J, Desvigne L, Lambros V, et al. Changes in ocular globe-to-orbital rim position with age: implications for aesthetic blepharoplasty of the lower eyelids. Aesthetic Plast Surg 1999; 23:337–342.
6. Zadoo V, Pessa J. Biological arches and changes to the curvilinear form of the aging maxilla. Plast Reconstr Surg 2000; 106:460–468.
7. Shaw RB Jr., Kahn DM. Aging of the midface bony elements: a three dimensional computed study. Plast Reconstr Surg 2007; 119:675–681.
8. Mittleman H. The anatomy of the aging mandible and its importance to face lift surger. Facial Plast Surg Clin North Am 1994; 2:301–311.
9. Rohrich R, Pessa JE. The fat compartments of the face: anatomy and clinical implications for cosmetic surgery. Plast Reconstr Surg 2007; 119(7):2219–2227.
10. Neuber F. Fat transplantation. Chir Konger Verhandl Dsch Gesellch Chir 1893; 20:66.
11. Lexer E. Correccion de los pechos dedulos (Mastroptose) por medio de la implantacian de grasa. San Sebastian Guipuzcoa Media 1921; 63:13. (Translated in Hinderer UT, del Rio JL, Erich Lexer's mammosplasty. Aesthetic Plast Surg 1992; 16:101–107).
12. Glashofer M, Lawrence N. Fat transplantation for treatment of the senescent face. Dermatol Ther 2006; 19:169–176.

13. Bruning P. (cited by Newman J, Ftaiha Z) The biographical history of fat transplant surgery. Am J Cosmet Surg 1987; 4:85.
14. Peer LA. Loss of weight and volume in human fat grafts. Plast Reconstr Surg 1950; 5:217–230.
15. Illouz YG. The fat cell "graft": a new technique to fill depressions. Plast Reconstr Surg 1986; 78:122–123.
16. Flynn TC, Coleman WP III, Field LM, et al. History of liposuction. Dermtol Surg 2000; 26:515–520.
17. Fournier PF. Facial recontouring with fat grafting. Dermatol Clin 1990; 8:523–537.
18. Fredricks S. Transplantation of purified autologuous fat: a three year follow-up is disappointing. Plast Reconstr Surg 1991; 87:228 (discussion).
19. Leever N. Cosmetic surgery—a comparison of its growth in the 1990s. Available at: http://www.cosmeticsurgery.org (compiled for the American Academy of Cosmetic Surgery). Accessed May 28, 2011.
20. Klein JA. Tumescent technique for regional anesthesia permits lidocaine dose of 35 mg/kg for liposuction. J Dermatol Surge Oncol 1990; 16:248–263.
21. Chajchi A, Benzaquen I. Fat-grafting injection for soft tissue augmentation. Plast Reconstr Surg 1989; 85:921–934.
22. Coleman SR. Facial recontouring with lipostructure. Clin Plast Surg 1997; 24: 347–367.
23. Pinski K, Roenigk H. Autologous fat transfer. Long-term follow-up. J Dermatol Surg Oncol 1992; 18:179–184.
24. Perez MI. Autologous fat transplantation: past and current practice. Cosmet Dermatol 1999; June:7–13.
25. Carpaneda CA, Riberio MT. Study of the histological alterations and viability of the adipose graft in humans. Aesthetic Plast Surg 1993; 17:43–47.
26. Sommer B, Sattler G. Current concepts of fat graft survival: histology of aspirated adipose tissue and review of the literature. Dermtol Surg 2000; 26:1159–1166.
27. Berman M. The aging face: a different perspective on pathology and treatment. Am J Cosmet Surg 1998; 15:167–172.
28. Fournier PM. Who should do syringe liposculpturing? J Dermatol Surg Oncol 1988; 14:1063–1073.
29. Guerrerosantos J. Simultaneous rhytidoplasty and lipoinjection: a comprehensive aesthetic surgical strategy. Plast Reconstr Surg 1998; 102:191–198.
30. Amar RE. Microinfiltration adipocytaire (MIA) auniveau de la face, ou recon-struction tissulaire par graffe de tissue adipeux. Ann Chirp Last Aesthet 1999; 44:593–608.
31. Donofrio LM. Fat distribution: a morphologic study of the aging face. Dermatol Surg 2000; 26:1107–1112.
32. Wesley NO, Dover JS. The filler revolution: a six year retrospective. J Drugs Dermatol 2009; 8(10):903–907.
33. Allan M, Dover JS. On beauty: evolution, psychosocial considerations and surgical enhancement. Arch Dermatol 2001; 137(6):795–807.
34. Robinson J, Anderson E. Skin structure and surgical anatomy. In: Robinson JK, Hanke CW, Sengelman RD, Siegal DM, eds. Surgery of the Skin. Philadelphia: Elsevier Mosby, 2005:3–23.
35. Hinderer UT. Malar implants for improvement of the facial appearance. Plast Reconstr Surg 1975; 56:157–165.

36. Wilkinson TS. Complications in aesthetic malar augmentation. Plast Reconstr Surg 1983; 71:643–649.
37. Silver WE. The use of alloplastic material in contouring the face. Facial Plast Surg 1986; 3:81–98.
38. Powell NB, Riley RW, Laub DR. A new approach to evaluation and surgery of the malar complex. Ann Plast Surg 1988; 20:206–214.
39. Prendergast M, Schoenrock LD. Malar augmentation. Patient classification and placement. Arch Otolaryngol Head Neck Surg 1989; 115:964–969.
40. Terino EO. Alloplastic facial contouring by zonal principles of skeletal anatomy. Clin Plast Surg 1992; 19:487–510.
41. Ellis DAF, Cousin JN. Surgical, injectable and synthetic lip enhancement. Otolaryngol Head Neck Surg 2000; 8:337–341.
42. Petrone A, Rizzi EB, Schinina V, et al. Sonographic assessment of facial HIV-related lipoatrophy. Dermatol Surg 2009; 35:1066–1072.
43. Vectra M3. Available at: http://www.canfieldsci.com. Accessed February 11, 2010.
44. Hudson DA, Lamber EV, Block CE. Site selection for autotransplantation. Some observations. Aesthetic Plast Surg 1990; 14:195.
45. Ullman Y, Hyams M, Ramon Y, et al. Enhancing the survival of the aspirated human fat injected into nude mice. Plast Reconstr Surg 1998; 101:1940–1944.
46. Rohrich RJ, Sorokin ES, Brown SA. In search of improved fat transfer viability: a quantitative analysis of the role of centrifugation and harvest site. Plast Reconstr Surg 2004; 113:391–395.
47. Moore J, Kolaczynski JW, Morales LM, et al. Viability of fat obtained by syringe suction lipectomy: effects of local anesthesia with lidocaine. Aesthetic Plast Surg 1995; 19:335–339.
48. Alexander RW, Maring TS, Aghabo T. Autologous fat grafting: a study of residual intracellular adipocyte lidocaine concentrations after serial rinsing with normal saline. Am J Cosmet Surg 1999; 16:123–126.
49. Keck M, Ueberreiter K, Janke J. Viability of preadipocytes in vitro: the influence of local anesthetics and the pH. J Dermatol Surg 2009; 35:1251–1257.
50. Fulton JE, Suarez M, Silverton K, et al. Small volume fat transfer. Dermtol Surg 1998; 24:857–865.
51. Lalikos J, Ya-Qi L, Roth T, et al. Biochemical assessment of cellular damage after adipocyte harvest. J Surg Res 1997; 70:95–100.
52. Chajchir A, Banzaquen I, Moretti E. Comparative experimental study of autologous adipose tissue processed by different techniques. Aesthetic Plast Surg 1993; 17:113–115.
53. Niechajev I, Sevuk O. Long-term results of fat transplantation: clinical and histological studies. Plast Reconstr Surg 1994; 94:496–506.
54. Jones JK, Lyles ME. The viability of human adipocytes after closed-syringe liposuction harvest. Am J Cosmet Surg 1997; 14:275–279.
55. Shiffman MA, Mirrafati S. Fat transfer techniques: the effects of harvest and transfer methods on adipocyte viability and review of the literature. Dermatol Surg 2001; 27:819–826.
56. Griffin EI. Results of fat transfer survey: criteria and interpretation. American Academy of Dermatology Annual Meeting, March 21, 1999; New Orleans, LA.
57. Johnson JG. Body contouring by microinjection of autogenous fat. Am J Cosmet Surg 1987; 16:248–262.

58. Kaufman MR, Bradley JP, Dickinson B, et al. Autologous fat transfer national consensus survey: trends in techniques for harvest, preparation, and application, and perception of short- and long-term results. Plast Reconstr Surg 2004; 113: 391–395.

59. Donofrio LM. Structural autologous lipoaugmentation: a pan-facial technique. Dermatol Surg 2000; 26:1129–1134.

60. Butterwick KJ. Lipoaugmentation for the aging hands: a comparison of the longevity and aesthetic results of centrifuged vs. non-centrifuged fat. Dermatol Surg 2002; 28:987–991.

61. Finder K. Personal communication. January 2001.

62. Available at: www.cytoritx.com/innovations/pipelineproducts.aspx#puregraft. Accessed January 11, 2010.

63. Shippert RD. Autologous fat transfer: eliminating the centrifuge, decreasing lipocyte trauma and establishing standardization for scientific study. Am J Cosmet Surg 2006; 23(1):21–27.

64. Moscatello DK, Schiavi J, Marquart JD, et al. Collagenase-assisted fat dissociation for autologous fat transfer. Dermatol Surg 2008; 34(10):1314–1322.

65. Hong SJ, Lee JH, Hong SM, et al. Enhancing the viability of fat grafts using new transfer medium containing insulin and beta-fibroblast growth factor in autologous fat transplantation. J Plast Reconstr Aesthet Surg 2010; 63(7):1202–1208.

66. Pallua N, Pulsfort AK, Suschek C, et al. Content of growth factors bFGF, IGF-1, VEGF and PDGF-BB in freshly harvested lipoaspirate after centrifugation and incubation. Plast Reconstr Surg 2009; 123:826–833.

67. Pinski KS. Fat transplantation and autologous collagen: a decade of experience. Am J Cosmet Surg 1999; 16:217–224.

68. Hernandez-Perez E, Lozano-Guarin JC. Fat grafting: techniques and uses in different anatomic areas. Am J Cosmet Surg 1999; 16:197–204.

69. Coleman WP III. Fat transplantation. Dermatol Clin 1998; 17:891–898.

70. Markey AC, Glogau RG. Autologous fat grafting: comparison of techniques. Dermatol Surg 2000; 26:1135–1144.

71. Shiffman MA. Effect of various methods of fat harvesting and reinjection. Am J Cosmet Surg 2000; 17:91–97.

72. Berman M. Rejuvenation of the upper eyelid complex with autologous fat transplantation. Dermatol Surg 2000; 26:1113–1116.

73. Amar RE. Fat autograft muscle injection. Presented at Association of Cosmetic Surgery Annual Meeting, February 2001; San Diego, CA.

74. Baran CN, Celbiogiu S, Sensoz O, et al. The behavior of fat grafts in recipient areas with enhanced vascularity. Plast Reconstr Surg 2002; 109:1646–1651.

75. Guerrerosantos J, Gonzalez-Mendoza A, Masmela Y, et al. Long-term survival of free fat grafts in muscle; an experimental study in rats. Aesthetic Plast Surg 1996; 20:403–408.

76. Zuk PA, Zhu M, Mizuno H, et al. Multi lineage cells from human adipose tissue: implications for cell based therapies. Tissue Eng 2001; 7(2):211–228.

77. Butterwick JK. Enhancement of the results of neck liposuction with the FAMI technique. J Drugs Dermtol 2003; 2:487–493.

78. Obagi S. The Obagi method of fat extraction, preparation, transplantation and follow-up. California Academy of Cosmetic Surgery, 11th Annual Conference. October 23–26, 2009.

79. Salasche SJ, Bernstein G, Senkarik M. Muscles of facial expression. In: Salasche SJ, Bernstein G, eds. Surgical Anatomy of the Skin. Norwalk, CT: Appleton & Lance, 1988:69–87.

80. Gray H. The facial muscles. In: Gross CM, ed. Anatomy of the Human Body. 107th ed. Philadelphia: Lea & Febiger, 1969:382–390.

81. Rose J, Lemke B, Lucarelle M, et al. Anatomy of facial recipient sites for autologous fat transfer. Am J Cosmet Surg 2003; 20:17–25.

82. Butterwick KJ. Fat autograft muscle injection (FAMI): new technique for facial volume. Dermatol Surg 2005; 31(11):1487–1495.

83. Butterwick KJ, Lack E. Facial volume restoration with fat autograft muscle injection (FAMI): preliminary experience with a new technique. Dermtol Surg 2003; 29:1019–1026.

84. Donofrio L. Technique of periorbital lipoaugmentation. Dermatol Surg 2003; 29:92–98.

85. Miller J, Popp J. Fat hypertrophy after autologous fat transfer. Ophthal Plast Reconstr Surg 2002; 18:228–231.

86. Bircoll M. Autologous fat transplantation: an evaluation of microcalcification and fat cell survivability following (AFT) cosmetic breast augmentation. Am J Cosmet Surg 1988; 5:283–288.

87. Har-Shai Y, Lindenbaum E, Ben-Itzhak O, et al. Large lipnecrotic pseudocyst formation following cheek augmentation by fat injection. Aesthetic Plast Surg 1996; 20:417.

88. Obagi S. Autologous fat augmentation and periorbital laser resurfacing complicated by abscess formation. Am J Cosmet Surg 2003; 20:155–157.

89. Dreizen NG, Framm L. Sudden unilateral visual loss after autologous fat injection in the glabellar area. Am J Ophthalmol 1989; 107:85–87.

90. Teimourian B. Blindness following fat injections. Plast Reconstr Surg 1988; 80:361.

91. Park SH, Sun HJ, Choi KS. Sudden unilateral visual loss after autologous fat injection into the nasolabial fold. Clin Ophthalmol 2008; 2(3):679–683.

92. Feinendegen D, Baumgartner R, Schroth G, et al. Middle cerebral artery occlusion and ocular fat embolism after autologous fat injection to the face. J Neurol 1998; 245:53–54.

93. Coleman SR. Avoidance of arterial occlusion from injection of soft tissue fillers. Aesthet Surg J 2002; 22:555–557.

94. Yoon SS, Chang DI, Chung KC. Acute fatal stroke immediately following autologous fat injection into the face. Neurology 2003; 61:1151–1152.

95. Wexler P. Tissue augmentation. Present and future. American Academy of Dermatology Annual meeting. March 2000; San Francisco, CA.

96. Coleman S. Complications of fat grafts and structural fillers. In: Techniques in minimally invasive aesthetic surgery. Los Angeles, 2002.

97. Horl HW, Feller AM, Biemer E. Technique for liposuction fat reimplantation and long-term volume evaluation by magnetic resonance imaging. Ann Plast Surg 1991; 26:248.

98. Goldman R, Carmargo CP, Goldman B. Fat transplantation and facial contour. Ann J Cosmet Surg 1998; 15:41–44.

99. Glogau RG. Microlipoinjection. Arch Dermatol 1988; 124:1340.

100. Fontdevila J, Serra-Renom J, Raigosa M, et al. Assessing the long-term viability of facial fat grafts: an objective measure using computed tomography. Aesthet Surg J 2008; 28(4):380–386.
101. Sadick NS, Hudgins LC. Fatty acid analysis of transplanted adipose tissue. Arch Dermatol 2001; 137:723–727.
102. Nguyen A, Pasyk KA, Bouvier TN, et al. Discussion: comparative study of survival of autologous adipose tissue taken and transplanted by different techniques. Plast Reconstr Surg 1990; 85:378–386.
103. Aboudib JHC Jr., deCastro CC, Gradel J. Hand rejuvenescence by fat filling. Ann Plast Surg 1992; 28:559–564.
104. Abrams HL, Lauber JS. Hand rejuvenation: the state of the art. Dermatol Clin 1990; 8:553–561.
105. Roh MR, Jung JY, Chung KY. Autologous fat transplant for depressed linear scleroderma-induced facial atrophic scars. J Dermatol Surg 2008; 34:1659–1665.
106. Eremia S, Newman N. Long-term follow up after autologous fat grafting: analysis of results from 116 patients followed at least 12 months after receiving the last of a minimum of two treatments. Dermatol Surg 2000; 26:1148–1158.
107. Perez M. Update on autologous fat transplantation. Cosmet Dermatol 2002; 15: 36–40.
108. Fournier PM. Fat grafting: my technique. Dermatol Surg 2000; 26:1117–1128.
109. Saylan Z. Frozen fat: better than fresh fat. Int J Cosmet Surg 1999; 7:39–42.
110. Takasu K, Takasu S. Long-term frozen fat transplantation. Int J Cosmet Surg 1999; 7:33–38.
111. Shoshani O, Ullmann Y, Shupak A, et al. The role of frozen storage in preserved adipose tissue obtained by suction-assisted lipectomy for repeated fat injection procedures. Dermatol Surg 2001; 27:645–647.
112. Butterwick KJ. Fresh versus frozen fat: a comparison of the longevity and aesthetic results for lipoaugmentation of the aging hands. Annual meeting of the American Society of Dermatologic Surgery. 2002; Chicago, IL.
113. MacRae JW, Tholpady SS, Ogle RC, et al. Ex vivo fat grafting preservation: effects and implications of cryopreservation. Ann Plast Surg 2004; 52(3):281–283.
114. Lawrence N. The science of fat transplantation. Advanced Cosmetic Seminar. Annual meeting of the American Society of Dermatologic Surgery. October 2002; Chicago, IL.
115. Moscatello DK, Dougherty M, Narins RS, et al. Cryopreservation of human fat for soft tissue augmentation: viability requires use of cryoprotectant and controlled freezing and storage. Dermatol Surg 2005; 31:1506–1510.
116. Pu LLQ, Cui X, Fink B, et al. Cryopreservation of adipose tissues: the role of trehalose. Aesthet Surg J 2005; 25:126–131.
117. Von Heimburg D, Zachariah S, Heschel I, et al. Human preadipocytes seeded on freeze-dried collagen scaffolds investigated in vitro and in vivo. Biomaterials 2001; 22:429–438.
118. Wang F, Garza L, Kang S, et al. In vivo stimulation of De Novo collagen production caused by cross-linked hyaluronic acid dermal filler injections in photo-damaged human skin. Arch Dermatol 2007; 143:155–163.
119. Carruthers J, Carruthers A. Facial sculpting and tissue augmentation. Dermatol Surg 2005; 31:1604–1612.

120. Vartanian AJ, Frankel AS, Rubin MG, et al. Injected hyaluronidase reduces restylane-mediated cutaneous augmentation. Arch Facial Plast Surg 2005; 7: 231–237.
121. Smith S, Busso M, McClaren M, et al. A randomized, bilateral, prospective comparison of calcium hydroxylapatite microspheres versus human-based collagen for the correction of nasalabial folds. Dermatol Surg 2007; 33:S112–S121.
122. Moers-Carpi M, Tufet JO. Calcium hydroxylapatite versus non-animal stabilized hyaluronic acid for the correction of nasolabial folds: a 12-month, multicenter, prospective, randomized, controlled, split-face trial. Dermtol Surg 2008; 34(2): 210–215.
123. Murray A, Zloty D, Warshawski L, et al. The evolution of soft tissue fillers in clinical practice. Dermatol Clin 2005; 23:343–363.
124. Hamilton T. Skin augmentation and correction: the new generation of dermal fillers—a dermatologist's experience. Clin Dermatol 2009; 27:S13–S22.
125. Butterwick KJ, Lowe N. Injectable PLLA for cosmetic enhancement: learning from the European experience. J Am Acad Dermatol 2009; 61(2):281–293.
126. Vleggaar D, Fitzgerald R. Dermatological implications of skeletal aging: a focus on supraperiosteal volumization for perioral rejuvenation. J Drugs Dermatol 2008; 7(3):209–220.
127. Swift A. Beauti "phi" cation: A mathematical analysis of beauty. In: Cosmetic Surgery Symposium. American Academy of Dermatology 67th Annual Meeting, March 6–10, 2009.
128. Mandy SH. What's new in fillers. Suppl Skin Aging 2009; 16–18.
129. Yoshimura K, Sato K, Aoi N, et al. Cell-assisted lipotransfer for facial lipoatrophy: efficacy of clinical use of adipose derived stem cells. Dermatol Surg 2008; 34: 1178–1185.

8

Cellulite pathophysiology and treatment

Andrei I. Metelitsa and Jaggi Rao

INTRODUCTION

Cellulite (also known as gynoid lypodistrophy, adiposis edematosa, dermo-panniculosis deformans, status protrusus cutis, edematous fibrosclerotic pan-niculopathy, atrophic panniculitis, and cellulitic hypodermosis) represents unaesthetic "cottage-cheese" or "orange peel" skin dimpling that is primarily observed in the gluteal-femoral regions of women, regardless of body shape and size (Fig. 8.1) (1,2). Given that it can be present in up to 98% of postpubertal women, some dermatologists have suggested that cellulite is part of normal female physiology and should not be treated like a disease (3). However, in today's culture, cellulite remains a subject of cosmetic concern for many patients who continue to request treatment solutions. Strong consumer demand has triggered the introduction of numerous treatment modalities with claims of complete eradication of cellulite, although comprehensive evidence-based clinical trials addressing the efficacy of such treatments are scarce. With even newer therapeutic approaches on the horizon, a thorough understanding of the etiologies, pathogenesis, and current treatment of this condition will allow clinicians to best counsel their patients.

BACKGROUND

In the earlier days, cellulite was often associated with beauty and attractiveness. The first description of cellulite was provided in the beginning of 19th century in French medical literature, when William Balfour first commented on the cutaneous nodule formation. More specific discussion of cellulite was provided in 1923 by French doctors Alquier and Paviot, who suggested that this unaesthetic condition was a result of noninflammatory dystrophy of mesenchymal tissue

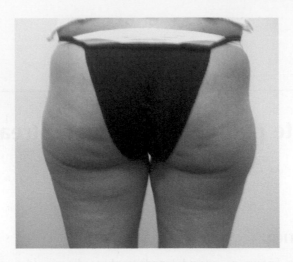

Figure 8.1   Typical anatomic sites of cellulite (buttocks and upper thighs).

characterized by interstitial fluid retention (4). Since then, a number of publications have provided new knowledge regarding cellulite pathophysiology and treatment (2,5–8).

CURRENT STATE OF KNOWLEDGE

Pathophysiology

It should be noted that a number of predisposing factors contribute to cellulite formation (Table 8.1). Although essentially every postpubertal woman develops some degree of cellulite, it is extremely uncommon in healthy men and is only apparent in individuals with androgen-deficient states. Cellulite should not be confused with obesity, with the latter showing only adipocyte hypertrophy and hyperplasia. In contradistinction, the pathogenesis of cellulite formation has been associated with a number of theories that include structural, vascular, and inflammatory changes (2,7,10).

Structural Theory

The theory of gender-related dimorphism has been proposed based on the identification of peculiar architectural extrusion of adipose tissue into the dermis that is characteristically seen in women. Herniated fat lobules, known as papillae adiposae, can protrude at the dermo-hypodermal interface, resulting in irregular and discontinuous surface and typical "pits" and "dells" of cellulite skin (5). These changes are not present in healthy male subjects who typically have

Table 8.1 Predisposing Factors for Cellulite Formation

Predisposing factors	Description
Gender	Cellulite occurs almost exclusively in women
Race	Cellulite is more common in Caucasian women than in Asian or African-American women
Heredity	Familial predisposition increases the likelihood of cellulite
Age	Cellulite is almost ubiquitous among postpubertal women
Increased subcutaneous fat	Greater adipose tissue in the subcutaneous layer enhances appearance of cellulite
Estrogen	Worsening of cellulite during pregnancy, nursing, menstruation
Emotional disturbance	Frustration, anxiety, depression, and stress can increase catecholamines and stimulate lipogenesis
Diet	High-fat diet can increase lipogenesis
Treatments	Estrogen therapy, antihistamines, antithyroid, β-blockers (9)

Source: From Refs. 7 and 11.

smooth and continuous dermo-hypodermal interface, accounting for gender-related structural characteristics (12). Given that papillae adiposae can also be found in clinically unaffected women (Fig. 8.2), additional factors are required to induce cellulite. A recent classification suggests separating cellulite into incipient or cellulite-prone stage versus full-blown cellulite (Table 8.2) (13). Gender-related dimorphism can account for incipient cellulite that is barely visible spontaneously, but can be demonstrated by the pinch test (14). Full-blown cellulite represents a more advanced form with lumpy-bumpy cutaneous cobbles

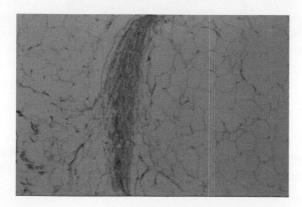

Figure 8.2 Histological section of cellulite-affected skin.

Table 8.2 Cellulite Classification

Grade I	No or minimal cellulite on observation; histopathology shows increased thickness of areolar layer and increased capillary permeability.
Grade II	Irregular skin topography on observation. Cellulite is enhanced by pinching or gluteal contraction. May have skin pallor, decreased temperature and sensation, and decreased elasticity.
Grade III	Skin exhibits classic *peau d'orange* appearance at rest. Small subcutaneous nodularities may be palpated.
Grade IV	More severe puckering, more palpable and painful nodules.

Source: From Refs. 7 and 11.

that can be distinctly observed on gross skin inspection (Figs. 8.3 and 8.4). Progression to full-blown cellulite results from continuous vertically oriented stretch within hypodermal collagen fibrous strands that is present in conjunction with the effect of gender-related dimorphism of the hypodermal connective tissue (14).

Vascular Theory

A proposed mechanism of cellulite formation has been outlined in the process of edematous fibrosclerotic panniculopathy (EFP) (8). In a series of triggering factors involving regional microcirculatory alterations, four evolutionary stages of EFP have been proposed. In response to alterations of the precapillary

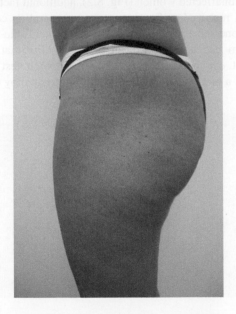

Figure 8.3 Appearance of mild-to-moderate cellulite (stage II).

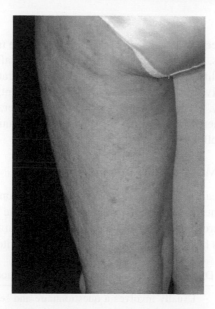

Figure 8.4 Appearance of moderate-to-severe cellulite (stage III).

arteriolar sphincter in affected areas, changes to capillary-venular permeability coupled with capillary ectasia result in retention of excess fluid within the dermis and interadipocyte septae (7). Increase in glycosaminoglycans in the dermis raises the interstitial pressure leading to further fluid retention (15). The resultant edema induces hypertrophy of the reticular fibers, which subsequently incorporate the adipocytes, and triggers micronodule formation. In the last stage of this process, sclerosis stimulates merging of micronodules, producing palpable macronodules that then induce visible surface irregularities on the skin.

Inflammatory Theory

Inflammatory changes resulting from collagen breakdown in the dermis may be responsible for fat herniation that leads to cellulite formation (3). Monthly menstrual cycles induce complex fluctuations in estrogen levels that are linked to the regulation of metalloproteases (MMPs), including MMP1 (collagenase), MMP2 (gelatinase A), and MMP9 (gelatinase B) (16,17). Estrogen-stimulated fibroblasts increase production of MMPs, thus leading to progressive damage in connective tissue via degradation of collagen fibers. The inflammatory nature of cellulite is also suggested by the association of gelatinase B with polymorphonuclear leukocytes, macrophages, and eosinophils (18), as well as presence of macrophages and lymphocytes in the fibrous septae of cellulite (19). The inflammation theory also explains subsequent worsening of cellulite with advancing age among postpubertal women following persistent collagen breakdown (3).

Treatment

Although there has been an increased level of interest in the treatment of cellulite over the recent years, no single method has been universally proven to be the best treatment modality. Presently, there are four basic categories of cellulite treatment: conservative management, topical management, injection therapy, and physical therapy. Adequate comparison of these therapies is often challenging given that there is a multitude of assessment techniques used to determine the extent of cellulite improvement (Table 8.3).

Conservative Management

Maintenance of a healthy lifestyle does not guarantee complete resolution of cellulite, but represents an important component of cellulite treatment. Ensuring a proper diet and exercise regimen may improve the appearance of the cellulite. Although weight loss has often been associated with cellulite reduction, in some

Table 8.3 Common Diagnostic Methods for Cellulite Evaluation

Patient self-assessment	Usually involves a questionnaire and self-rated visual analogue scales
Observer evaluation	(*i*) *Direct visualization* of cellulite with further assessment of puckering, dimpling, and nodularities; manual palpation ideally performed in a dark room with tangential lighting
	(*ii*) *Standardized photography* with proper illumination at reproducible position (20)
Anthropometry	*Body mass index* (BMI) = person's weight in kilograms divided by height in meters squared; does not correlate directly with cellulite
	Circumference (mainly thigh)—indirect measure of cellulite (varies with edema, trauma, exercise, activity)
Skin elasticity	Measures skin tension with a suction elastometer to determine resilience of the dermis
Ultrasound (US)	Noninvasive, readily available imaging technique that allows visualization of the dermo-hypodermal tissue interface.
Magnetic resonance imaging (MRI)	Noninvasive, visualization of dermo-hypodermal interface, further assessment of adipose tissue with its high-resolution coronal slices (21,22)
Histopathology	Invasive, specific method of evaluating the histological extent of cellulite; does not always correlate with clinical appearance
Laser Doppler flowmetry	Assessment of skin microcirculation (23)
Thermography	Indirect measure of blood flow through the assessment of skin surface; rarely used (24)

women it may actually worsen the appearance of cellulite. In a study assessing the effect of weight loss on cellulite appearance among 62 women, a bimodal distribution in response was documented (25). The majority of the patients who improved were found to have a higher body mass index. The authors concluded that relatively minor weight loss coupled with a less compliant (looser) skin at baseline can negatively influence cellulite appearance during weight loss.

Although these lifestyle modifications cannot eliminate cellulite completely, they may reduce the clinical appearance of skin puckering by decreasing adipocyte volume.

Topical Management

Although numerous topical agents, including xanthines, retinoids, lactic acid, and herbals are available to the consumer, the application of these agents for the purpose of cellulite treatment remains questionable (26). Mechanisms of action include promotion of lipolysis, stimulation of collagen deposition, and increase of microvascular flow and lymphatic drainage (11). Review of published data shows that the most successful topical agent incorporates multiple active anti-cellulite ingredients.

Topically applied methylxanthines, including caffeine, aminophylline, theobromine, and theophylline, are biologic phosphodiesterase inhibitors that can increase cyclic adenosine monophosphate (cAMP) and are thought to stimulate lipolysis (27). Topical caffeine, one of the most commonly used additives in anticellulite preparations is thought to improve vascular and lymphatic flow through vasodilation and lipolysis (28). In a two-center, double-blinded, randomized trial of 40 women, the effect of a four-week daily application of a novel topical agent that contained caffeine as one of its active ingredients was studied, and evaluation of photographs by dermatologists revealed cellulite improvement in 68% of subjects (11). The average measured decrease in thigh circumference was 1.93 cm with the active product and 1.27 cm with a placebo. When combined with retinol and ruscogenine in an alcohol vehicle, topical caffeine was effective in improving skin texture as was demonstrated in a three-month double-blind evaluation of 46 women (23).

Preliminary studies on aminophylline, despite showing improvement, have either lacked controls (29) or showed very minimal changes (30). A prospective, 12-week randomized controlled study showed no evidence for the use of aminophylline in cellulite treatment, given that only 3 of the 35 treated patients claimed improvement on self-evaluation (31).

Topical retinoids have been suggested to potentially restrict the herniation of the fat tissue into the dermis by thickening the dermis through the promotion of the synthesis of glycosaminoglycans and increasing the deposition of collagen in the dermis. Two main studies have so far investigated the effect of topical retinol in the treatment of cellulite, but their relevance remains to be seen. In a double-blind study that involved 20 women, topical 0.3% retinol was applied twice daily on one thigh and placebo vehicle on the other thigh for a period of six months (32). Of the 19 subjects, 13 rated the retinol side as more improved, with a 0.16-mm increase in ultrasound (US)-measured dermal thickness on the retinol side and a significant increase in blood flow measurements. Furthermore, another randomized, placebo-controlled study involving 15 women who applied topical retinol daily for six months on thighs did not show any improvement in overt cellulite, although certain characteristics of incipient cellulite were felt to be improved (33). The authors noted a 10.7% increase in skin elasticity and 15.8% decrease in viscosity and were able to demonstrate a two- to fivefold increase in the number of factor XIIIa+ dendrocytes both in the dermis and in fibrous strands of the hypodermis. These changes may ultimately improve resting tensions inside the skin leading to smoother surface, but the evidence remains inconclusive.

Although lactic acid, an α-hydroxy acid, has been studied in the treatment of cellulite based on its possible effect on improving the stratum corneum, there is no proof of its clinical efficacy (34).

Despite the availability of numerous topical herbal treatments containing specific mixtures of botanical extracts with claims of anticellulite properties, clinical significance remains unclear (Table 8.4) (1).

Injection Therapy

Mesotherapy is a technique that involves intra- or subcutaneous injection of a mixture of therapeutic compounds for a variety of conditions, including reduction of fat and cellulite (35). Multiple substances, including vasodilators, anti-inflammatory agents, vitamins, minerals, plant extracts, hormones, antibiotics, enzymes, coenzymes, and anesthetics, have been used in combination with this technique (36). Mesotherapy proponents claim that it enhances circulation and lymphatic drainage and stimulates β-adrenoreceptors on the adipocyte cell surface, which increases lipolysis (36). Lipolysis, induced by mesotherapy substances including isoproterenol, aminophylline, yohimbine, and melilotus, may then have the potential to improving cellulite appearance.

Injection lipolysis with sodium deoxycholate used alone or in combination with phosphatidylcholine offers promising application in fat reduction and possible utility in cellulite treatment (37). A detailed discussion of these agents and their associated techniques is provided in chapter 6.

Physical Therapies

Massage/Endermologie. Lymphatic drainage is a massage technique that is performed in the direction of lymphatic return and is designed to reduce the stasis of lymphatic fluid and stimulate lymphatic flux. If performed appropriately, it can lead to thinning of the subcutaneous fat and improvement in cellulite appearance (38).

Table 8.4 Herbal Extracts Used in the Treatment of Cellulite

Herbal name	Parts of the plant	Main constituents	Mechanism of action
Bladderwrack	Whole dried thallus	Sulfated polysaccharides, iodine compounds, alginic acid	Increases density of dermal connective tissue
Butcher's broom	Rhizome, flowering tops	Saponins, ruscogenin, neororuscogenin	Increase microvascular flow
Centella asiatica	Leaves, roots	Asiaticoside, madecassic acid, asiatic acid	Increase microvascular flow
Chofitol or artichoke	Leaves, flower heads, roots	Enzymes, cynarin, ascorbic acid, caffeoylquininc acid derivatives, flavonoids	Increase microvascular flow
Common Ivy	Leaves, stems	Flavonoids, saponins	Increase microvascular flow
Corynarth yohimbe, Pausinystalia youhimbe, and Rauwolfia serpentina	Leaves, shells, roots	Yohimbe; alpha-yohimbine	Reduce lipogenesis and promote lipolysis
Ginkgo	Leaves	Flavinoids, biflavons, terpenes	Destroy free-radical formation
Ground Ivy	Leaves, stems	Flavonoids, triterpenoids, phenolic acids	Increase microvascular flow
Indian or horse chestnut	Seeds, shells	Triterpenoid saponins, flavones, coumarins, tannins	Increase microvascular flow
Papaya and pineapple	Fruits, leaves	Papain, bromelain	Increase microvascular flow
Red grapes	Skin, stems, seeds	Tannins, procianidins	Destroy free-radical formation
Sweet Clover	Flowers, leaves	Coumarin	Increase microvascular flow

Source: From Ref. 1.

Endermologie represents a newer technique that involves a patented machine-assisted massage system consisting of two rollers designed to suction the skin. Originally developed in France, LPG Endermologie (LPG Systems, Valence, France)—also known as skin kneading—received FDA approval in 1998 for temporary reduction in the appearance of cellulite. This therapy increases blood and lymphatic flow and thus improves the underlying fat-tissue architecture. More recently, increased lipolytic responsiveness of adipose tissue was found following treatment with this technique (39). In a one-year clinical outcome study of Endermologie in 85 patients, 46 patients completed 7 treatment sessions and 39 patients completed 14 treatment sessions (40). The former group showed a mean index reduction of 1.34 cm in body circumference, whereas the latter group showed a reduction of 1.83 cm and 90% of the patients reported favorable improvements in their cellulite-affected areas. Another 12-week prospective, randomized, controlled trial included twice-weekly Endermologie treatment with or without aminophylline cream (31). Although 10 of the 35 Endermologie-treated patients reported that their cellulite appearance improved, the authors did not feel that this was an effective treatment for cellulite because of marginal results. A recent study of 33 women treated with Endermologie showed mild reduction in cellulite grade in only five patients (41).

Ultrasound. High-frequency US has been used in hydrolipoclasia, a procedure for the treatment of fat and cellulite that induces degeneration of adipocytes via injection of physiologic solution into subdermal tissue followed by ultrasonic massage (7).

Noninvasive US devices have recently been evaluated for body contouring applications. Medsculpt (Alderm, Irvine, California, U.S.) and Dermosonic (Symedex, Minneapolis, Minnesotta, U.S.) are FDA-approved devices for cellulite reduction that incorporate vacuum suction and massage (42). Another device, Ultrashape (Ultrashape Ltd., Tel Aviv, Israel), emits focused US waves to deliver concentrated mechanical energy into subcutaneous tissue and to induce lipolysis. A prospective study of 30 patients who underwent 3 monthly treatment sessions with Ultrashape demonstrated a mean decrease of 2.3 cm in fat thickness and a circumference reduction of 4.0 cm (43). Definitive, larger studies are still required to properly assess these treatment modalities.

Radio frequency. A number of new noninvasive radio frequency (RF) devices that have been studied over the past several years have shown not only potential but also innovation with regards to cellulite treatment. Given excellent safety profiles, these devices include the VelaSmooth (Syneron Medical Ltd., Yokneam, Israel), Accent (Alma Lasers, Buffalo Grove, Illinois, U.S.), Thermalipo (Thermamedic Ltd., Alicante, Spain), and TriPollar (Regen, Pollogen Ltd., Tel Aviv, Israel). The mode of action of RF devices in cellulite is thought to be related to skin tightening through the heating of dermis and subcutaneous tissues, collagen contraction, and subsequent formation of new collagen fibers, as well as possible lipolysis (44,45).

Velasmooth, approved by the FDA in 2005 for the treatment of cellulite, is a device that utilizes bipolar RF, infrared (IR) light (700–2000 nm), and mechanical massage with suction (750 mmHg of negative pressure). This system uses vacuum suction and massage from mechanical rollers to increase local blood supply to the adipose tissue and, subsequently, to increase oxygen availability. Mechanical manipulation of tissue also promotes lymphatic drainage. Additional delivery of IR light and the bipolar RF, two different ranges of electromagnetic energy, supplies the heat that facilitates fat metabolism through a theoretical increase in the available oxygen (46).

A prospective report on the efficacy and safety of this technology described 35 women with cellulite on thighs and/or buttocks who received 8 to 16 twice-weekly treatments (46). Most of the patients had mild-to-moderate improvement in cellulite appearance when rated by physicians and a mean reduction of 2 cm in thigh circumference, although no histological changes were noted between treated and untreated sites (46). Another study of 20 women with moderate bilateral thigh and buttock cellulite who received eight twice-weekly treatments showed approximately 50% clinical improvement, with circumferential thigh reduction of 0.8 cm on the treatment side (47). A smaller subsequent study of 10 women investigating results of 12 treatment sessions also showed more than 25% visual improvement in cellulite in half of the treated subjects (48). Specific histological changes in the affected buttocks of 10 women before and two hours after a single treatment with Velasmooth were also recently assessed (49). Although no thermal damage was noted in the epidermis or dermis, changes related to incipient necrosis were found in the subcutaneous tissue, with adipocytes showing alteration in physical integrity and signs of membrane lysis (49). Frequency of treatment sessions still needs to be established and, although a small prospective noted visible clinical improvement one year after the last treatment (50), most of the investigators agree that once-monthly maintenance treatments should be implemented to enhance results (47,51).

Thermalipo is a novel bipolar device that utilizes automatic multi-frequency and low impedance (AMFLI) RF. This technology allows rapid deposition of high energy load without the need for epidermal cooling (52). In a multicenter study of cellulite treatment involving 50 women who received 12 once-weekly sessions, patient satisfaction index of 76% and physician-assessed overall efficacy of 66% were noted (52). A slight decrease in efficacy was reported two months after the treatment, suggesting the need for maintenance sessions similar to other RF technologies. Histological findings from 30 biopsies taken immediately after a single Thermalipo session showed polyhedral and rectangular adipocytes with evidence of membrane degeneration, reduced or no lipid content, and apoptotic changes (53).

Accent, a unipolar RF device, received FDA approval for the treatment of cellulite in 2009. This device produces high-frequency electromagnetic radiation allowing effective heating of deeper structures when compared to bipolar devices. One of the initial studies of this device involved US evaluation of 26 patients with visible bilateral cellulite on either the buttock and/or thighs who received two treatments sessions (54). The authors noted an approximate 20% volume contraction among 68% of the patients; however, no cellulite assessment was performed. Another cohort of 30 women with upper-thigh cellulite received six treatments every other week (55). Twenty-seven of the subjects showed evidence of clinical improvement with a mean decrease of 2.45 cm in leg circumference and a graded improvement of 2.9 on a scale of 1 to 4, with 4 being the highest. Additional histological evidence of posttreatment dermal fibrosis was also demonstrated. It should be noted that a smaller study of 10 patients with thigh cellulite treated at similar parameters showed a mean overall cellulite improvement of only 8% and no statistical significance was noted (56).

TriPollar is a novel RF device, which utilizes three electrodes (one positive pole and two negative poles). This allows for simultaneous heating of the superficial and deep skin layers, theoretically combining the effects of mono- and bipolar RF (57). Advantages of this technology include high power density, deep penetration depth, and no requirement of skin cooling (57). Following eight once-weekly treatment sessions in 37 women, blinded investigators noted approximately 50% improvement in cellulite appearance with significant circumference reduction of 3.5 and 1.7 cm in the abdomen and thigh regions, respectively (57). This technology, similar to other RF modalities, has been shown to induce increased dermal thickness because of focal thickening of collagen fibers (58).

Lasers and light sources. Intense pulse light (IPL) emits light in the visible and near-IR spectrum and has been found to stimulate collagen production (59). A 12-week course of treatment using Quadra Q4 IPL (DermaMed, Media, Pennsylvania, U.S.) in combination with a compounded retinyl-based cream, demonstrated more than 50% improvement in cellulite at three months, with less visible effects in the IPL-only group (60). US evaluations of selected patients in the study demonstrated increased collagen deposition in the cellulite areas.

A combination treatment consisting of a light-emitting diode (LED) device emitting red and near-IR light (660 nm and 950 nm, respectively) and phosphatidylcholine-based topical anticellulite gel has been also suggested to reduce cellulite (61). Possible mechanisms of LED action include stimulation of procollagen synthesis, downregulation of MMP-1 activity, and anti-inflammatory action. Following 24 twice-weekly LED sessions and twice-daily cream application for three months, eight of the nine thighs were downgraded to a lower cellulite grade by clinical examination and photography. Given that relapses were noted between 6 and 15 months after the treatment, the authors emphasized the importance of maintenance treatments.

TriActive (Cynosure Inc., Chelmsford, Massachusetts, U.S.), approved by the FDA in 2004 for the treatment of cellulite, is a device that employs a low-energy diode laser (810 nm) and tissue massage. Its treatment effect in cellulite reduction is thought to be based on the combined action of mechanical massage to increase lymphatic drainage, localized cooling to counter any burning sensation, and deep laser penetration to stimulate collagen production and tighten the skin. In a clinical trial involving 16 patients, 21% improvement in cellulite was noted after 12 twice-weekly treatments (62). In a separate single-center, randomized, comparative, prospective study of 20 patients, both Tri-Active and VelaSmooth provided 25% improvement in cellulite with no statistically significant difference between the devices (63).

GentleYAG (Candela Corp., Wayland, Massachusetts, U.S.), a long-pulsed Nd:YAG laser with a wavelength of 1064 nm, has also been studied in the treatment of cellulite because of its ability to deeply penetrate the skin, to induce bulk heating of the deep dermis, and to stimulate fibroblasts to produce new collagen. Three treatments with high fluence of 30 J/cm^2 and spot size of 18 mm have been shown to induce skin tightening in one study of 12 patients, although an ultrasonic and a photographic examination of treated areas showed only slight improvement in the appearance of cellulite (64).

Smoothshapes (Elemé Medical, Merrimack, New Hampshire, U.S.), approved by the FDA in 2006 for the reduction of cellulite, features proprietary Photomology technology, which synergistically combines electromagnetic energy, including that from a 915-nm laser and a 650-nm light source, with mechanical manipulation—contoured rollers for massage and vacuum suctioning. Thus, the 915-nm laser specifically targets and liquefies fat, the 650-nm light increases cell membrane permeability, which allows liquefied fat to enter lymphatic circulation, and the contoured rollers and vacuum facilitate movement of fat and promote lymphatic drainage. In a study of 74 individuals who completed 14 treatment sessions with this device over four to six weeks, an MRI assessment showed a reduction in fat thickness by 1.19 cm^2 on the treated leg, with 82.26% of patients responding to treatment; however, no specific cellulite assessment measurements were discussed (65).

Subcision.   Subcision is a simple surgical technique, which has been proposed as a treatment of moderate-to-high grade of cellulite (66,67). It is performed using a special scalpel or an 18-gauge Nokor Admix needle (Becton Dickinson, Franklin Lakes, New Jersey, U.S.), which is inserted into subcutaneous tissue in a repetitive motion parallel to the epidermis. At the level of subcutaneous fat, this technique is thought to have three mechanisms of action, including shearing of fat septae, formation of new connective tissue, and subsequent redistribution of fat and tensile forces between the lobes (67). In a three-year study of 232 patients with clinically apparent cellulite, this procedure was found to be successful in 79% of patients who were satisfied with their improvements (67). Postoperatively, however, all patients developed pain, bruising, and hyperpigmentation. This study's limitations included lack of a control group and the subjective nature of the assessment.

Injections of preserved particulate fascia coupled with subcision may be more effective than subcision alone. In a small series of eight women with a total of 56 cellulite depressions on the thighs, 91% of the depressions showed improvement following this combination approach (68). Larger studies will be necessary to corroborate these findings.

Liposculpture/liposuction. Although liposuction has been considered in the treatment of cellulite, documented improvement is often minimal. The theoretical reduction in cellulite appearance occurs as a result of decreased fat volume as well as disruption of fibrous bands that are associated with skin dimpling. Several techniques are available, including traditional liposuction, tumescent liposuction, ultrasound-assisted liposuction, and laser lipolysis (69). These techniques are described in detail elsewhere in this book.

A combination of laser lipolysis utilizing subdermal Nd:YAG laser and autologous fat transplantation has been recently investigated in a study of 52 women with advanced cellulite (70). Laser lipolysis under tumescent conditions was combined with autologous fat injections to the most depressed areas. The majority of treated patients subjectively rated their cellulite improvement to be more than 50%; however, no objective measurements were provided in the study.

Miscellaneous therapies. The following therapeutic modalities have also been suggested for the treatment of cellulite; however, some have since been disproved, while others still require further clinical confirmation of their effectiveness.

Extracorporeal pulse activation therapy. Extracorporeal pulse activation therapy (EPAT), also known as extracorporeal acoustic wave therapy, is a noninvasive therapy that utilizes slow-intensity acoustic waves and pulses with the intent of potentially improving cellulite. A recent analysis of 59 women with advanced cellulite revealed strengthening of the connective tissue and a 73% increase in skin elasticity at the end of the treatment (71).

Carboxytherapy. Carboxytherapy involves therapeutic use of carbon dioxide (CO_2) via transcutaneous or subcutaneous injection. Known to improve circulation and tissue perfusion, this therapy has also been shown to induce fracturing of adipose tissue and has thus been advocated for the treatment of localized adiposities and cellulite (72,73).

Pressotherapy. Pressotherapy is a noninvasive lymphatic drainage treatment that uses inflating pumps to create intermittent pneumatic compression (7). This system employs five compression chambers that are positioned around the limbs and focus on increasing venous and lymphatic flow. This technique has been used as an adjunctive therapy for cellulite, for example, in combination with Endermologie. However, the results have been discouraging (41).

Iontophoresis. Iontophoresis involves generation of electromagnetic field through the application of galvanic current on the skin. One of the mechanisms of treatment is based on the current's vasomotor action, which leads to vasodilation and may generate metabolic changes, which can then enhance the appearance of cellulite. Its true efficacy in cellulite reduction, however, still needs to be shown; therefore, this therapy is not presently recommended.

Thermotherapy. Thermotherapy is a technique that involves induction of vasodilation by applying heat. However, this technique may also potentially aggravate cellulite since high temperature is known to cause protein denaturation (7).

CONCLUSIONS

Over the past several years, a number of new, mostly minimally invasive interventions have been advocated in the treatment of cellulite. Although some treatments selectively target adipocytes to induce lipolysis, others provide a permanent camouflage by thickening collagen in the dermis. At this stage, no single treatment can offer complete eradication of cellulite. However, innovative approaches will continue to push the field to address this extremely common esthetic concern. Until then, careful assessment of existing evidence and possible combination treatments that incorporate several existing modalities will ensure maximized efficacy.

REFERENCES

1. Hexsel D, Orlandi C, Zechmeister do Prado D. Botanical extracts used in the treatment of cellulite. Dermatol Surg 2005; 31:866–872.
2. Avram MM. Cellulite: a review of its physiology and treatment. J Cosmet Laser Ther 2004; 6:181–185.
3. Draelos ZD. The disease of cellulite. J Cosmet Dermatol 2005; 4:221–222.
4. Alquier L. La cellulite. In: Sergent E, Ribadeau-Dumas L, Babonneix L, eds. Traité de Pathologie Médicale et de Thérapcutique Appliquée. Paris: Maloine et Fils Editeurs, 1924:533–552.
5. Nurnberger F, Muller G. So-called cellulite: an invented disease. J Dermatol Surg Oncol 1978; 4:221–229.
6. Scherwitz C, Braun-Falco O. So-called cellulite. J Dermatol Surg Oncol 1978; 4:230–234.
7. Rossi AB, Vergnanini AL. Cellulite: a review. J Eur Acad Dermatol Venereol 2000; 14:251–262.
8. Curri SB. Cellulite and fatty tissue microcirculation. Cosmet Toilet 1993; 108.51–58.
9. Ciporkin H, Paschoal LH. Atalizaçã Terapêutica e Fisiopatogênica Da Lipodistrofia Ginóide (LDG) "Celullite." São Paulo: Livraria Editora Santos, 1992.

10. Terranova F, Berardesca E, Maibach H. Cellulite: nature and aetiopathogenesis. Int J Cosmet Sci 2006; 28:157–167.
11. Rao J, Gold MH, Goldman MP. A two-center, double-blinded, randomized trial testing the tolerability and efficacy of a novel therapeutic agent for cellulite reduction. J Cosmet Dermatol 2005; 4:93–102.
12. Rosenbaum M, Prieto V, Hellmer J, et al. An exploratory investigation of the morphology and biochemistry of cellulite. Plast Reconstr Surg 1998; 101: 1934–1939.
13. Pierard GE. Commentary on cellulite: skin mechanobiology and the waist-to-hip ratio. J Cosmet Dermatol 2005; 4:151–152.
14. Quatresooz P, Xhauflaire-Uhoda E, Pierard-Franchimont C, et al. Cellulite histopathology and related mechanobiology. Int J Cosmet Sci 2006; 28:207–210.
15. Lotti T, Ghersetich I, Grappone C, et al. Proteoglycans in so-called cellulite. Int J Dermatol 1990; 29:272–274.
16. Singer CF, Marbaix E, Lemoine P, et al. Local cytokines induce differential expression of matrix metalloproteinases but not their tissue inhibitors in human endometrial fibroblasts. Eur J Biochem 1999; 259:40–45.
17. Curry TE Jr., Osteen KG. The matrix metalloproteinase system: changes, regulation, and impact throughout the ovarian and uterine reproductive cycle. Endocr Rev 2003; 24:428–465.
18. Jeziorska M, Nagase H, Salamonsen LA, et al. Immunolocalization of the matrix metalloproteinases gelatinase B and stromelysin 1 in human endometrium throughout the menstrual cycle. J Reprod Fertil 1996; 107:43–51.
19. Kligman AM. Cellulite: facts and fiction. J Geriatr Dermatol 1997; 5:136–139.
20. Bielfeldt S, Buttgereit P, Brandt M, et al. Non-invasive evaluation techniques to quantify the efficacy of cosmetic anti-cellulite products. Skin Res Technol 2008; 14: 336–346.
21. Mirrashed F, Sharp JC, Krause V, et al. Pilot study of dermal and subcutaneous fat structures by MRI in individuals who differ in gender, BMI, and cellulite grading. Skin Res Technol 2004; 10:161–168.
22. Hexsel DM, Abreu M, Rodrigues TC, et al. Side-by-side comparison of areas with and without cellulite depressions using magnetic resonance imaging. Dermatol Surg 2009; 35:1471–1477.
23. Bertin C, Zunino H, Pittet JC, et al. A double-blind evaluation of the activity of an anti-cellulite product containing retinol, caffeine, and ruscogenine by a combination of several non-invasive methods. J Cosmet Sci 2001; 52:199–210.
24. Vasallo C, Berardesca E. Efficacy of a multifunctional plant complex in the treatment of a localized fat-lobular hypertorphy. Am J Cosmet Surg 2001; 18:203–208.
25. Smalls LK, Hicks M, Passeretti D, et al. Effect of weight loss on cellulite: gynoid lypodystrophy. Plast Reconstr Surg 2006; 118:510–516.
26. van Vliet M, Ortiz A, Avram MM, et al. An assessment of traditional and novel therapies for cellulite. J Cosmet Laser Ther 2005; 7:7–10.
27. Draelos ZD, Marenus KD. Cellulite. Etiology and purported treatment. Dermatol Surg 1997; 23:1177–1181.
28. Sainio EL, Rantanen T, Kanerva L. Ingredients and safety of cellulite creams. Eur J Dermatol 2000; 10:596–603.
29. Artz JS, Dinner MI. Treatment of cellulite deformities of the thighs with topical aminophylline gel. Can J Plast Surg 1995; 3:190–192.

30. Hamilton EC, Greenwawy FL, Bray GA. Regional fat loss from the thigh in women using 2% aminophylline. Obesity Res 1993; 1:95S.

31. Collis N, Elliot LA, Sharpe C, et al. Cellulite treatment: a myth or reality—a prospective randomized, controlled trial of two therapies, endermologie and aminophylline cream. Plast Reconstr Surg 1999; 104:1110–1114; discussion 5–7.

32. Kligman AM, Pagnoni A, Stoudemayer T. Topical retinol improves cellulite. J Dermatol Treat 1999; 10:119–125.

33. Pierard-Franchimont C, Pierard GE, Henry F, et al. A randomized, placebo-controlled trial of topical retinol in the treatment of cellulite. Am J Clin Dermatol 2000; 1:369–374.

34. Smith WP. Cellulite treatments: snake oils or skin science. Cosmet Toilet 1995; 110: 61–70.

35. Pistor M. What is mesotherapy? Chir Dent Fr 1976; 46:59–60.

36. Rotunda AM, Kolodney MS. Mesotherapy and phosphatidylcholine injections: historical clarification and review. Dermatol Surg 2006; 32:465–480.

37. Rotunda AM, Weiss SR, Rivkin LS. Randomized double-blind clinical trial of subcutaneously injected deoxycholate versus a phosphatidylcholine-deoxycholate combination for the reduction of submental fat. Dermatol Surg 2009; 35:792–803.

38. Bayrakci TV, Akbayrak T, Bakar Y, et al. Effects of mechanical massage, manual lymphatic drainage and connective tissue manipulation techniques on fat mass in women with cellulite. J Eur Acad Dermatol Venereol 2010; 24:138–142.

39. Monteux C, Lafontan M. Use of the microdialysis technique to assess lipolytic responsiveness of femoral adipose tissue after 12 sessions of mechanical massage technique. J Eur Acad Dermatol Venereol 2008; 22:1465–1470.

40. Chang P, Wiseman J, Jacoby T, et al. Noninvasive mechanical body contouring: (Endermologie) a one-year clinical outcome study update. Aesthetic Plast Surg 1998; 22:145–153.

41. Gulec AT. Treatment of cellulite with LPG endermologie. Int J Dermatol 2009; 48: 265–270.

42. Foster KW, Kouba DJ, Hayes J, et al. Reductions in thigh and infraumbilical circumference following treatment with a novel device combining ultrasound, suction, and massage. J Drugs Dermatol 2008; 7:113–115.

43. Moreno-Moraga J, Valero-Altes T, Riquelme AM, et al. Body contouring by non-invasive transdermal focused ultrasound. Lasers Surg Med 2007; 39:315–323.

44. Alster TS, Tehrani M. Treatment of cellulite with optical devices: an overview with practical considerations. Lasers Surg Med 2006; 38:727–730.

45. Alexiades-Armenakas M. Laser and light-based treatment of cellulite. J Drugs Dermatol 2007; 6:83–84.

46. Sadick NS, Mulholland RS. A prospective clinical study to evaluate the efficacy and safety of cellulite treatment using the combination of optical and RF energies for subcutaneous tissue heating. J Cosmet Laser Ther 2004; 6:187–190.

47. Alster TS, Tanzi EL. Cellulite treatment using a novel combination radiofrequency, infrared light, and mechanical tissue manipulation device. J Cosmet Laser Ther 2005; 7:81–85.

48. Sadick N, Magro C. A study evaluating the safety and efficacy of the VelaSmooth system in the treatment of cellulite. J Cosmet Laser Ther 2007; 9:15–20.

49. Trelles MA, Mordon SR. Adipocyte membrane lysis observed after cellulite treatment is performed with radiofrequency. Aesthetic Plast Surg 2009; 33:125–128.

50. Wanitphakdeedecha R, Manuskiatti W. Treatment of cellulite with a bipolar radio-frequency, infrared heat, and pulsatile suction device: a pilot study. J Cosmet Dermatol 2006; 5:284–288.

51. Romero C, Caballero N, Herrero M, et al. Effects of cellulite treatment with RF, IR light, mechanical massage and suction treating one buttock with the contralateral as a control. J Cosmet Laser Ther 2008; 10:193–201.

52. van der Lugt C, Romero C, Ancona D, et al. A multicenter study of cellulite treatment with a variable emission radio frequency system. Dermatol Ther 2009; 22:74–84.

53. Trelles MA, van der Lugt C, Mordon S, et al. Histological findings in adipocytes when cellulite is treated with a variable-emission radiofrequency system. Lasers Med Sci 2010; 25:191–195.

54. Emilia del Pino M, Rosado RH, Azuela A, et al. Effect of controlled volumetric tissue heating with radiofrequency on cellulite and the subcutaneous tissue of the buttocks and thighs. J Drugs Dermatol 2006; 5:714–722.

55. Goldberg DJ, Fazeli A, Berlin AL. Clinical, laboratory, and MRI analysis of cellulite treatment with a unipolar radiofrequency device. Dermatol Surg 2008; 34:204–209; discussion 9.

56. Alexiades-Armenakas M, Dover JS, Arndt KA. Unipolar radiofrequency treatment to improve the appearance of cellulite. J Cosmet Laser Ther 2008; 10:148–153.

57. Manuskiatti W, Wachirakaphan C, Lektrakul N, et al. Circumference reduction and cellulite treatment with a TriPollar radiofrequency device: a pilot study. J Eur Acad Dermatol Venereol 2009; 23:820–827.

58. Kaplan H, Gat A. Clinical and histopathological results following TriPollar radiofrequency skin treatments. J Cosmet Laser Ther 2009; 11:78–84.

59. Goldberg DJ. New collagen formation after dermal remodeling with an intense pulsed light source. J Cutan Laser Ther 2000; 2:59–61.

60. Fink JS, Mermelstein H, Thomas A, et al. Use of intense pulsed light and a retinyl-based cream as a potential treatment for cellulite: a pilot study. J Cosmet Dermatol 2006; 5:254–262.

61. Sasaki GH, Oberg K, Tucker B, et al. The effectiveness and safety of topical Pho-toActif phosphatidylcholine-based anti-cellulite gel and LED (red and near-infrared) light on grade II-III thigh cellulite: a randomized, double-blinded study. J Cosmet Laser Ther 2007; 9:87–96.

62. Boyce S, Pabby A, Chuchaltkaren P, et al. Clinical evaluation of a device for the treatment of cellulite: Triactive. Am J Cosmet Surg 2005; 22:233–237.

63. Nootheti PK, Magpantay A, Yosowitz G, et al. A single center, randomized, comparative, prospective clinical study to determine the efficacy of the VelaSmooth system versus the Triactive system for the treatment of cellulite. Lasers Surg Med 2006; 38:908–912.

64. Bousquet-Rouaud R, Bazan M, Chaintreuil J, et al. High-frequency ultrasound evaluation of cellulite treated with the 1064 nm Nd:YAG laser. J Cosmet Laser Ther 2009; 11:34–44.

65. Lach E. Reduction of subcutaneous fat and improvement in cellulite appearance by dual-wavelength, low-level laser energy combined with vacuum and massage. J Cosmet Laser Ther 2008; 10:202–209.

66. Orentreich DS, Orentreich N. Subcutaneous incisionless (subcision) surgery for the correction of depressed scars and wrinkles. Dermatol Surg 1995; 21:543–549.

67. Hexsel DM, Mazzuco R. Subcision: a treatment for cellulite. Int J Dermatol 2000; 39:539–544.
68. Burres S. Correcting cellulite with preserved particulate fascia injections. Cosmet Dermatol 2005; 18:141–144.
69. Igra H, Satur NM. Tumescent liposuction versus internal ultrasonic-assisted tumescent liposuction. A side-to-side comparison. Dermatol Surg 1997; 23: 1213–1218.
70. Goldman A, Gotkin RH, Sarnoff DS, et al. Cellulite: a new treatment approach combining subdermal Nd: YAG laser lipolysis and autologous fat transplantation. Aesthet Surg J 2008; 28:656–662.
71. Christ C, Brenke R, Sattler G, et al. Improvement in skin elasticity in the treatment of cellulite and connective tissue weakness by means of extracorporeal pulse activation therapy. Aesthet Surg J 2008; 28:538–544.
72. Brandi C, D'Aniello C, Grimaldi L, et al. Carbon dioxide therapy in the treatment of localized adiposities: clinical study and histopathological correlations. Aesthetic Plast Surg 2001; 25:170–174.
73. Brandi C, D'Aniello C, Grimaldi L, et al. Carbon dioxide therapy: effects on skin irregularity and its use as a complement to liposuction. Aesthetic Plast Surg 2004; 28:222–225.

9

Future technologies, trends, and techniques

Jennifer Chwalek and Alexander L. Berlin

INTRODUCTION

As shown in the previous chapters, a multitude of therapeutic options are currently available for the treatment of disorders of fat and cellulite. Although some modalities have been around for decades, others are just now becoming available. Propelling these developments is a desire for a perfect treatment: one with consistent, excellent results with no or little downtime and no adverse effects or complications. Although no such treatment is available at this time, the demand for one has lead to a number of innovations in the field.

One exciting feature of this quest for advancements in technologies and techniques is the variety of approaches to the same problem. Thus, improvements continue to be made to the time-tested procedures, such as liposuction, as well as to some newer techniques, such as energy-based therapeutic modalities, as in the case of cryolipolysis.

Although future trends and innovations are always difficult to predict, this chapter will present some recent developments in the field of fat and cellulite.

FUTURE TECHNOLOGIES AND TECHNIQUES

Stem Cells and Autologous Fat Transfer

As mentioned in chapter 7, adipose-derived stem cells (ASCs) have emerged as an important contributor to cell viability and, ultimately, successful volume correction (1). Recently, microencapsulation using alginate powder has been tried in an animal model. Both in vitro and in vivo experiments using mice showed durable clinical improvement, as well as increased cell survival and lower donor cell migration (2). Microencapsulation was accomplished using an electrostatic bead generator, a relatively simple procedure that may have the potential of being easily integrated into an office setting. So far, no studies involving human subjects have been performed using this technique.

Staged stem cell–enriched tissue injections have recently been studied, especially in the context of difficult recipient areas, such as those occurring in hemifacial atrophy, burn scars, and previously irradiated tissue (3). In the process, traditional autologous fat grafting is followed on the same day by the injection of fat grafts enriched with adipose-derived regenerative cells (ADRCs). ADRCs are comprised of adipose stem cells, as well as angiogenic and other progenitor cells. This stepwise process is thought to contribute to better cell viability and graft survival because of proangiogenic and antiapoptotic action by the ADRCs.

Platelet-Rich Plasma

Although platelet concentrates have been around for more than a decade, their integration into clinical practice has been slow. Several factors have been responsible for that, including specialized equipment requirements, additional expense associated with the procedure, and lack of commercially available kits. Lately, this technique has been significantly simplified with the emergence of several devices that can quickly and easily concentrate and activate platelets.

Platelet-rich plasma (PRP) is prepared from a small amount of autologous blood, which is then subjected to a slow centrifugation at $1100g$. This process leads to the precipitation of erythrocytes and leukocytes at the bottom of the centrifuge tube, with platelets being suspended in the supernatant plasma. Platelets are then activated using divalent calcium, resulting in degranulation (4).

Platelet α granules contain a large number of growth factors, cytokines, and chemokines, including transforming growth factors (TGF) α and β, epidermal growth factor, vascular endothelial growth factor, platelet-derived growth factor, insulin-like growth factor, fibrinogen, fibronectin, thrombospondin, osteocalcin, osteonectin, and others (5,6). Many of these factors are involved in clotting and subsequent wound healing (7).

PRP may be used alone or, more commonly, in combination with autologous fat grafting. It has been shown that PRP significantly increases the number of ASCs—three- to fourfold—and results in enhanced graft survival over time, including in patients with facial diseases, such as hemifacial atrophy (4). Furthermore, the addition of a fibrin matrix improves the release of platelet-derived growth factors and leads to a further increase in graft survival and terminal differentiation of preadipocytes (8–10). A device that facilitates the production of autologous platelet-rich fibrin matrix (PRFM) (Selphyl, Aesthetic Factors, LLC, Princeton, New Jersey, U.S.) has recently been introduced into the market and has been dubbed in the media as the "vampire facelift."

Additional large prospective studies will be needed to establish clinical relevance of these techniques. Future studies may also reveal their applicability to the healing process following some of the other procedures described in this book.

Three-Dimensional Scaffolds and Adipose Tissue Engineering

The previously mentioned strategies of microencapsulation and fibrin matrices are only two examples of the numerous developments in adipose tissue engineering. Armed with a better understanding of the complex physiological processes underlying the differentiation of ASCs and preadipocytes into mature adipocytes, vascular proliferative factors, and other necessary components of a conducive microenvironment, bioengineers have been developing a variety of three-dimensional scaffold structures. Such tissue scaffolds provide physical support, as well as protective boundary conditions, for developing tissue. In order for such three-dimensional constructs to be clinically relevant, they need to be histioinductive; that is, they need to induce neovascularization and recruit resident stem cells (11). Finally, they need to be biocompatible and degradable in vivo to eventually be completely replaced by host tissue.

Numerous natural and synthetic materials have been studied for adipose tissue engineering. Some of the examples of engineered structures include polyethylene glycol–based hydrogels; woven and nonwoven polyester meshes; electrospun nanofibrous matrices; synthetic polymer or silk fibroin three-dimensional porous scaffolds; as well as hyaluronic acid, collagen, and cross-linked gelatin sponges (12–18). Most investigations, however, have so far only been conducted either in vitro or in animal models. Nonetheless, the sheer number of developments in this field is very encouraging and future studies may confirm potential clinical applications for some of these approaches.

Novel Injectable Agents and Delivery Modes

The demand for noninvasive treatment options has resulted in the development of a variety of topical products for cellulite, most of which contain methylxanthines or phosphodiesterase inhibitors that modulate cell lipolysis. As mentioned in chapter 8, these topical preparations have produced unremarkable results because of insufficient dermal penetration. Employing these drugs through the use of iontophoresis or mesotherapy may, however, result in significant transdermal concentrations to be of clinical relevance in the future (19). In addition, newer drug delivery systems employing nanotechnology, microneedle arrays, ultrasound, radiofrequency, and laser irradiation have shown varying degrees of promise.

Novel cryopneumatic and photopneumatic technologies have been studied in *ex porcine* and in vivo human skin models to enhance hydrophilic percutaneous drug delivery. Through freezing and stretching the skin with vacuum suction, cryopneumatic technology creates small openings in the skin allowing for more direct delivery of medications. Likewise, photopneumatic technology also creates microcuts in the skin with vacuum suction, but instead of freezing uses intense pulse light (20). Since many of the treatments for cellulite and fat disorders discussed in this book use energy-based technology, combining these devices with topical or injectable substances for more efficient drug delivery and to maximize responses will likely become the next therapeutic milestone. However, the pharmokinetics and safety of infusible treatments will need to be carefully studied.

As mentioned in chapter 8, carboxytherapy is another example of a novel injectable treatment that has shown promise for localized adiposities and cellulite. Transcutaneous infiltration of CO_2 appears to cause microcirculatory changes in fat because of the Bohr effect and the resulting increased oxygenation of CO_2-laden tissue. Increased tissue perfusion following carboxytherapy has been confirmed with Doppler flowmetry and transcutaneous measurement of oxygen tension (21). Clinical improvement following five sessions of carboxytherapy to the thigh was demonstrated in a study of 57 women at the two-week follow-up visit. This was accompanied by histological evidence of lipolysis and dermal thickening (21,22). However, whether this treatment can result in any lasting improvement needs to be determined in future studies.

As our understanding of fat metabolism evolves, newer fat-altering substances are being explored. Subcutaneous botulinum neurotoxin A has shown a lipolytic effect in rabbits, presumably through interference with cholinergic innervation (23). Flavonoids and hormones such as leptin are other injectable agents that have resulted in reduced subcutaneous fat in animal studies (24,25). Their clinical role in injection lipolysis remains to be seen.

Energy-Based Technologies

Advances in energy-based treatments for fat and cellulite will probably involve modifications of current devices and, most likely, combinations of different modalities. For instance, radiofrequency (RF), as described in the previous chapters, has the unique advantage of targeting subcutaneous tissue and creating bulk tissue heating with little to no epidermal effect. Recent studies have examined the use of RF devices capable of targeting different tissue planes with more selective volumetric heating based on the anatomical area treated. Although these devices are still too slow to be of practical significance, newer generations of RF devices with tunable operational frequencies will allow the operator to selectively treat larger volumes of fat faster (26,27).

As mentioned in chapter 8, acoustic wave therapy (AWT) or extracorporeal pulse activation therapy (EPAT) is another technology still in its nascent stages of development for cutaneous and subcutaneous disorders. This technique has previously been used in lithotripsy of renal and urethral calculi as well as in the healing of musculoskeletal disorders such as fractures. EPAT utilizes low-amplitude acoustic waves of long duration to create local tissue damage and to improve blood circulation. It has also been shown to induce lipolysis and to stimulate collagen production (28–31). In addition, upregulation of signaling proteins, such as vascular endothelial growth factor (VEGF) and endothelial nitric oxide synthase (eNOS), and an increase in the level of tissue antioxidants have been noted following EPAT. A study of 59 women with moderate to severe cellulite treated with EPAT for three to four weeks revealed increased skin elasticity and more compact connective tissue as measured by ultrasound. Results persisted and even improved by the six-month follow-up visit (29). Another study of 25 women consisted of six AWT sessions over four weeks and measured three-dimensional skin textural changes as outcome criteria. Statistically significant improvement was noted in treated versus untreated skin in regard to depressions, elevations, roughness, and elasticity. This improvement lasted up to three months following the last session (28). Thus, although most of the previously discussed technologies have noted changes in circumference as a measure for reduced adipose tissue, this therapy may also be successful in treating textural changes associated with cellulite.

Gene Targeted Therapy

One of the most exciting areas of development that will likely impact therapeutic options for adipose tissue is the genetics and physiology of lipid metabolism and cellulite. Recently, Emanuele et al. demonstrated angiotensin-converting enzyme (ACE) and hypoxia inducible factor 1 alpha (HIF1A) polymorphisms in lean women with cellulite (32). Their work supports the idea that local circulatory dysregulation and reduced blood perfusion may have a critical role in the pathogenesis of cellulite. There is also evidence that angiotensin II can be produced locally in adipose tissue (32). Adipogenesis and obesity may result in increased angiotensin II because of increased secretion of angiotensinogen by adipocytes. There is speculation that dysregulation of these local hormones results in reduced blood flow to adipose tissue, adipocyte hyperplasia, edema, and altered extracellular matrix architecture (32).

As mentioned in chapter 2, there are many other genes that have been identified and found to be involved in adipocyte regulation. Medications that modulate these genes or their products may help to prevent or halt the progression of cellulite or fat disorders. For instance, the cannabinoid-1 receptor (CB-1) is present in the feeding regions of the brain as well as in adipocytes. Rimonabant, a selective CB-1 receptor blocker, has been studied for its effects on satiety and weight loss. Preliminary trials showed it successfully increased weight loss and reduced waist circumference (33). Although the side effects of rimonabant precluded clinical application, other CB-1 receptor antagonists are still being examined. Peroxisome proliferator–activated receptor (PPAR) agonists, such as thiazolidinediones, increase peripheral insulin sensitivity and are used to treat diabetes. The PPAR agonists also promote extracellular matrix production and skin tightening (34). Other medications that indirectly stimulate PPARs, such as salicylates and fibrates, may have a role in improving adipocyte function (33).

Perilipin and adiponectin are hormones that have pivotal roles in fat catabolism (33–36). Coptis root extract has been shown to reduce gene expression of perilipin and increase lipolysis of arterial plaques in atherosclerosis-prone mice (35). Increased adiponectin levels, which inversely correspond to body fat levels, have been seen following bariatric surgery and the administration of several pharmacological agents, including statins, aldosterone antagonists, and metformin. Direct administration of adiponectin may also be a potential treatment for fat disorders if a biologically active form of the molecule is developed. These are just a few examples of possible pharmacological targets that may revolutionize the way we approach adipocyte disorders.

CONCLUSIONS

Spurred at least in part by the new research into the physiology of adipose tissue, the field of fat and cellulite treatments is expected to continue to grow rapidly in the foreseeable future. Such developments will likely result in safer and more efficacious therapeutic modalities.

REFERENCES

1. Yoshimura K, Sato K, Aoi N, et al. Cell-assisted lipotransfer for facial lipoatrophy: efficacy of clinical use of adipose derived stem cells. Dermatol Surg 2008; 34: 1178–1185.
2. Moyer HR, Kinney RC, Singh KA, et al. Alginate microencapsulation technology for the percutaneous delivery of adipose-derived stem cells. Ann Plast Surg 2010; 65(5):497–503.
3. Tiryaki T, Findikli N, Tiryaki D. Staged stem cell-enriched tissue (SET) injections for soft tissue augmentation in hostile recipient areas: a preliminary report. Aesthetic Plast Surg April 13, 2011 [Epub ahead of print].
4. Cervelli V, Gentile P, Scioli MG, et al. Application of platelet-rich plasma in plastic surgery: clinical and in vitro evaluation. Tissue Eng Part C Methods 2009; 15(4):625–634.
5. Sclafani AP. Applications of platelet-rich fibrin matrix in facial plastic surgery. Facial Plast Surg 2009; 25(4):270–276.
6. Cervelli V, Palla L, Pascali M, et al. Autologous platelet-rich plasma mixed with purified fat graft in aesthetic plastic surgery. Aesthetic Plast Surg 2009; 33(5): 716–721.
7. Anitua E, Andia I, Ardanza B, et al. Autologous platelets as a source of proteins for healing and tissue regeneration. Thromb Haemost 2004; 91(1):4–15.
8. Anitua E, Sanchez M, Nurden AT, et al. Autologous fibrin matrices: a potential source of biological mediators that modulate tendon cell activities. J Biomed Mater Res A 2006; 77(2):285–293.

9. Torio-Padron N, Baerlecken N, Momeni A, et al. Engineering of adipose tissue by injection of human preadipocytes in fibrin. Aesthetic Plast Surg 2007; 31(3): 285–293.

10. Schoeller T, Lille S, Wechselberger G, et al. Histomorphologic and volumetric analysis of implanted autologous preadipocyte cultures suspended in fibrin glue: a potential new source for tissue augmentation. Aesthetic Plast Surg 2001; 25(1): 57–63.

11. Tanzi MC, Fare S. Adipose tissue engineering: state of the art, recent advances and innovative approaches. Expert Rev Med Devices 2009; 6(5):533–551.

12. Alhadlaq A, Tang M, Mao JJ. Engineered adipose tissue from human mesenchymal stem cells maintains predefined shape and dimension: implications in soft tissue augmentation and reconstruction. Tissue Eng 2005; 11(3-4):556–566.

13. Kang X, Xie Y, Powell HM, et al. Adipogenesis of murine embryonic stem cells in a three-dimensional culture system using electrospun polymer scaffolds. Biomaterials 2007; 28(3):450–458.

14. Lamme EN, Druecke D, Pieper J, et al. Long-term evaluation of porous PEGT/PBT implants for soft tissue augmentation. J Biomater Appl 2008; 22(4):309–335.

15. Mauney JR, Nguyen T, Gillen K, et al. Engineering adipose-like tissue in vitro and in vivo utilizing human bone marrow and adipose-derived mesenchymal stem cells with silk fibroin 3D scaffolds. Biomaterials 2007; 28(35):5280–5290.

16. Rhodes NP, Bartolo CD, Hunt JA. Analysis of the cellular infiltration of benzyl-esterified hyaluronan sponges implanted in rats. Biomacromolecules 2007; 8(9): 2733–2738.

17. von Heimburg D, Kuberka M, Rendchen R, et al. Preadipocyte-loaded collagen scaffolds with enlarged pore size for improved soft tissue engineering. Int J Artif Organs 2003; 26(12):1064–1076.

18. Lin SD, Wang KH, Kao AP. Engineered adipose tissue of predefined shape and dimensions from human adipose-derived mesenchymal stem cells. Tissue Eng Part A 2008; 14(5):571–581.

19. Altabas K, Altabas V, Berkovic MC, et al. From cellulite to smooth skin: is Viagra the new dream cream? Med Hypotheses 2009; 73:118–125.

20. Sun F, Anderson R, Aguilar G. Stratum corneum permeation and percutaneous drug delivery of hydrophilic molecules enhanced by cryopneumatic and photopneumatic technologies. J Drugs Dermatol 2010; 9(12):1528–1530.

21. Lee GSK. Carbon dioxide therapy in the treatment of cellulite: an audit of clinical practice. Aesthetic Plast Surg 2010; 34:239–243.

22. Brandi C, D'Aniello C, Grimaldi L, et al. Carbon dioxide therapy in the treatment of localized adiposities: clinical study and histopathological correlations. Aesthetic Plast Surg 2001; 25:170–174.

23. Bagheri M, Jahromi BM, Bagheri M, et al. A pilot study on the lipolytic effect of subcutaneous botulinum toxin injection in rabbits. Anal Quant Cytol Histol 2010; 32(4):186–191.

24. Zarrouki B, Pillon NJ, Kalbacher E, et al. Cirsimarin, a potent antilipogenic flavonoid, decreases fat deposition in mice intra-abdominal adipose tissue. Int J Obes 2010; 34(11):1566–1575.

25. Donahoo WT, Stob NR, Ammon S, et al. Leptin increases skeletal muscle lipoprotein lipase and postprandial lipid metabolism in mice. Metabolism 2011; 60(3):438–443.

26. Franco W, Kothare A, Goldberg DJ. Controlled volumetric heating of subcutaneous adipose tissue using a novel radiofrequency technology. Lasers Surg Med 2009; 41: 745–750.

27. Franco W, Kothare A, Ronan SJ, et al. Hyperthermic injury to adipocyte cells by selective heating of subcutaneous fat with a novel radiofrequency device: feasibility studies. Lasers Surg Med 2010; 42:361–370.

28. Adatto M, Adatto-Neilson R, Servant JJ, et al. Controlled, randomized study evaluating the effects of treating cellulite with AWT/EPAT. J Cosmet Laser Ther 2010; 12:176–182.

29. Christ C, Brenke R, Sattler G, et al. Improvement in skin elasticity in the treatment of cellulite and connective tissue weakness by means of extracorporeal pulse activation therapy. Aesthet Surg J 2008; 28(5):538–544.

30. Reddy BY, Hantash BM. Emerging technologies in aesthetic medicine. Dermatol Clin 2009; 27(4):521–527.

31. Angehrn F, Kuhn C, Voss A. Can cellulite be treated with low-energy extracorporeal shock wave therapy? Clin Interv Aging 2007; 2(4):623–630.

32. Emanuele E, Bertona M, Geroldi D. A multilocus candidate approach identifies ACE and HIF1A as susceptibility genes for cellulite. J Eur Acad Dermatol Venereol 2010; 24:930–935.

33. Westerink J, Visseren FLJ. Pharmacological and non-pharmacological interventions to influence adipose tissue function. Cardiovasc Diabetol 2011; 10(1):13.

34. Khan MH, Victor F, Rao B, et al. Treatment of cellulite: Part II. Advances and controversies. J Am Acad Dermatol 2010; 62(3):373–384.

35. Zhou MX, Xu H, Chen KJ, et al. Effect of Coptis root extract on gene expressions of perilipin and PPAR-gamma in aortic vulnerable atherosclerotic plaque of ApoE-gene knockout mice. Zhongguo Zhong Xi Yi Jie He Za Zhi 2008; 28(6):532–536.

36. Yamauchi T, Kamon J, Minokoshi Y, et al. Adiponectin stimulates glucose utilization and fatty-acid oxidation by activating AMP-activated protein kinase. Nat Med 2002; 8(11):1288–1295.

10

Clinical management of the patient

Lori Brightman and Robert Anolik

INTRODUCTION

The consumer demand for cosmetic procedures continues to rise, with reportedly more than eight million body-shaping procedures performed in 2008 (1). The demand has grown in part because of the expanding number of cosmetic procedures available, particularly those with reproducible efficacy and limited downtime. This is most evident in the field of body contouring. For many years, the only option for those seeking improvement in the cosmetic appearance of the body was surgical. Now, technological advances have brought about the arena of noninvasive and minimally invasive approaches. These options are important to help meet the demands of patients who are not surgical candidates, prefer not to undergo surgical procedures, do not have the needed downtime, or are not comfortable with the associated surgical risks.

BACKGROUND

The clinical management of a patient presenting with body shape concerns is widely divergent based on a number of factors. One must consider demographics, such as age, sex, genetics, and overall health. In addition, intended goals, tolerance of downtime, and acceptance of procedural risk will influence management options. Specific concerns must be clarified, since certain anatomic locations may favor a particular method of intervention. Similarly, unwanted characteristics within an area, such as skin laxity as opposed to fat volume, may call for other interventions. The multitude of factors influencing management must be understood to establish realistic expectations and yield a satisfied patient.

When managing the patient, the physician ought to consider all treatment options. Although each patient encounter is distinct and, therefore, firm algorithms cannot be fixed, Figure 10.1 highlights several of the minimally invasive

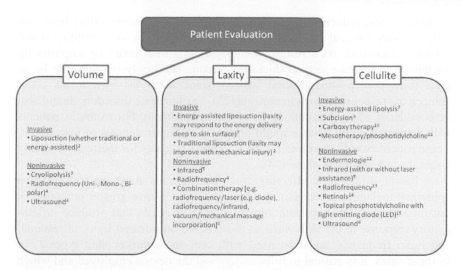

Figure 10.1 Minimally invasive and noninvasive strategies based on principal concern.

and noninvasive strategies based on specific complaints, namely volume, laxity, and cellulite (2-15).

CLINICAL MANAGEMENT

Patient Characteristics: Age, Sex, and Race

A patient's age may influence which approach is recommended. In many ways, this is logical, as a more surgical approach, such as tumescent liposuction, might yield longer recovery periods and more risk for infection considering the relative cardiovascular and immunologic compromise in older patients. One would also consider the likelihood of ideal results being achieved in a more senior patient. For example, an older patient may experience less than ideal skin retraction after liposuction and, therefore, be left with less than desirable results (16).

Concerns for age may also influence the choice of noninvasive therapies, since other, less well-understood factors may likely contribute to the treatment results. For example, infrared or radio frequency contouring devices are designed to trigger inflammatory and wound-healing responses with subsequent neocollagenesis (17). However, inflammation and collagen development may be sparse in older patients, as literature highlights differences in skin and fibroblast-like skin cells at older ages (18–20).

Sex of the patient also plays a role in the approach to patients, since gender differences in the skin have been recognized in dermatology (21). These differences include epidermal and dermal thickness along with weight distribution and reduction (22). How these differences might affect treatment efficacy with surgical or noninvasive treatments for fat and cellulite is not entirely understood. As a result, technologies that treat laxity or adiposity by attempting to increase dermal thickness or stimulate lipolysis might not be an ideal therapy in postmenopausal women, since lower estrogen levels could dampen the response to such treatments (23). Sex hormone disorders should also be considered when determining the course of treatment. For example, patients with polycystic ovary disease might present with higher degrees of visceral fat. These patients would therefore not be suitable candidates for therapies that only target the subcutaneous plane (24).

Racial differences affecting treatment options most notably involve epidermal melanin concentrations. Darker skin types have greater potential for postinflammatory dyspigmentation. As a result, devices that produce inflammatory response in the skin, such as those based on infrared light, ultrasound, and radio frequency, must be used with caution in darker skin types (25). In these cases, it is critical to fully understand the device employed and which parameters would allow an effective treatment yet would still be safe for a darker skin type.

Physical Examination

Medical Conditions

A small percentage of patients present for a body contouring consultation with medical concerns. In these cases, treatment is geared toward the specific area of pathology. Examples include lipomas; angiolipomas; gynecomastia; and less commonly encountered lipodystrophy conditions such as Madelung disease, Dercum disease, and Barraquer–Simons syndrome, among others. Depending on the severity of pathology, some of these patients may be relatively more motivated for treatment and emotionally equipped to endure the discomfort of the more aggressive approaches. However, the etiology or progression of these pathologies ought to be considered in the management of the patient. For example, if a simple lipoma has developed without any other medical history, a patient may strongly desire laser lipolysis, as this could help avoid an obvious scar from a surgical excision. However, when faced with more unusual situations, such as Barraquer–Simons syndrome, in which a patient might develop lower-body fat hypertrophy, one should ask whether intervention would prove futile if hypertrophy rapidly redevelops.

Baseline Examination

Investigation into the patient's overall health status is imperative for optimal results in all patients. One would begin by inquiring about past medical history, current medications and known drug allergies, weight fluctuation, prior

Table 10.1 Contraindications of Various Treatment Approaches

Invasive and noninvasive approaches in general	Pregnancy
	Active infection in treatment area
	Severe comorbidities (e.g., cardiovascular compromise or uncontrolled diabetes)
	History of abnormal healing
Radio frequency	Pacemaker/defibrillator
	Metal implants below or near the treatment area
Cryolipolysis	Cryoglobulinemia
	Paroxysmal cold hemoglobulinuria
	Cold urticaria
Laser	Photosensitive disorders such as lupus and porphyria
	Medications or supplements that produce photosensitivity such as isotretinoin, tetracycline, ciprofloxacin, diltiazem, furosemide
	Tattoo or permanent ink in the treatment area
	Tanned skin
Mesotherapy/ phosphotidylcholine (with or without LED)	Allergy to the various injectables (methylxanthines, such as caffeine, aminophylline, theophylline; hormones; enzymes; herbal extracts; vitamins; minerals; phosphotidylcholine)
	If LED is incorporated into phosphotidylcholine treatment, patients ought not have photosensitive disorders or take photosensitizing medications
Topical herbs and retinols	Allergy to these agents
	Pregnancy in instances of retinol use

procedures in the intended treatment area, scars, and any medical conditions. History and physical examination might reveal evidence for poor wound healing, such as hypertrophic scars or keloids. Medications and allergies should be reviewed extensively, as anticoagulants may affect even minimally invasive approaches, resulting in the increased risk of bleeding and ecchymoses, and allergies can affect the choice of anesthetics and perioperative pharmaceuticals. Other health concerns should also be thoroughly examined, in particular for invasive procedures, such as vascular status, the use of tobacco, diet, and exercise. There are also general and treatment-dependent contraindications to therapy (Table 10.1).

Patient Selection

Patient selection is one of the most critical steps in delivering optimal results. A challenge for many physicians arises when a patient has a particular procedure in

mind because of second-hand stories—a friend's experience or coverage of a
new device in the media. It is the responsibility of the physician to understand a
patient's principal concern and motivation and then both acknowledge their
particular inquiries and explain why their suggestion may or may not be best
suited for their condition. For example, a postbariatric patient would likely have
significant skin redundancy and would be best suited for plasty procedures rather
than noninvasive skin-tightening procedures. Furthermore, a patient who is
seeking fat volume reduction and is significantly over his or her optimal body
mass index (BMI) is not a good candidate for cryolipolisis (26).

A patient presenting for body contouring who reports a history of multiple
prior procedures, dissatisfaction with prior cosmetic procedures, significant
weight fluctuation, or who has unrealistic goals may have emotional or psychological instability or even more severe conditions, such as body dismorphic
syndrome. It is vital to recognize these issues so that the patient can be properly
cared for from a psychiatric standpoint. Moreover, when treated despite psychiatric illness, these patients tend to have a low satisfaction rate and can be
potentially medically and legally problematic.

Weight, nutrition, and exercise should also be directly addressed during the
consultation. The ideal candidate is close to his or her target body mass index
and has a healthy diet and exercise regimen in place yet experiences resistant
pockets of fat or skin laxity. If a patient is steadily increasing in weight, or
chooses to not adhere to a balanced diet and is mostly sedentary, procedural
intervention may have limited benefit (27).

In addition to the patient characteristics listed previously, specific
patient concerns play a critical role in management. Of the different treatment
options discussed at length in this book, some work better for certain areas
than others. For example, lipohypertrophy concentrated in the "love handles"
or lower abdomen might respond well to liposuction or cryolipolysis.
However, if addressing laxity in the lower abdomen, infrared or radio
frequency would be a more appropriate choice. Also, in some circumstances,
more than one procedure or a combination of treatments may be best for the
ideal results.

Body Contouring Treatments

Just as important as patient selection, the individual treatment itself needs to
be well understood to optimize its efficacy against a target area and specific
circumstance. This is best illustrated by radio frequency systems. Energy
output for a particular device is directly related to the current, impedance, and
time (28). This is described in Joule's law, $J = I^2 \times z \times t$, where J is energy, I
is current, z is impedance, and t is time in seconds. Lack et al. demonstrated
that impedance varies with anatomic area and is based on the composition of
anatomic structures, such as dermis, fat, muscle, and bone (29). Impedance

was highest on the dorsal arm and lowest on the back in this study. Appreciation of the impedance levels at each area of treatment may allow the practitioner a better sense of energy output per anatomic region and potential degree of effect.

Upon patient evaluation, the fat-to-laxity ratio in the target area also plays a key role in determining the optimal treatment option. When lipohypertrophy is the primary concern, liposuction or cryolipolysis might serve as the best option for the patient. When textural laxity is the principal concern, other options using radio frequency, infrared light, suction, and massage may offer better option. It is important to note here that when considering a treatment device that employs suction, some degree of tissue laxity is required. This laxity allows the tissue to be easily manipulated into the device hand piece to deliver an ideal treatment. This could be a challenge when treating areas with limited laxity such as over bone or over muscular areas of an athlete.

Patient Expectations

Perhaps the most important step in patient management is setting realistic expectations. This often requires a thorough consultation of all options, discussion of potential side effects, and the signing of an informed consent that not only highlights potential benefits but also complications. During such detailed consultations, patients might reveal unrealistic or unreasonable expectations, such as avoiding a divorce or gaining a promotion from improving their shape. By establishing what may or may not be achieved, there is a far greater chance of having a satisfied patient.

When discussing expectations, it is valuable for patients to understand that results may fall within a certain range and that where they find themselves afterward is somewhat unpredictable. This discussion could include an explanation of the different fat types (visceral and subcutaneous), skin laxity, and degrees of variability in response in different patients and in different anatomic locations of the same individual.

Baseline Documentation

A valuable management tool in all cosmetic patients is the use of baseline documentation to demonstrate posttreatment enhancement (Table 10.2). Improvement, especially subtle, as can be achieved with some contouring treatments, may be difficult to appreciate for the patient herself. Traditional methods for documenting baseline status for fat and cellulite concerns have included standard two-dimensional photographs and tape measurements. However, advances in measurement devices have followed suit with body-shaping devices. These include laser levels as well as objective three-dimensional imaging systems that can quantifiably demonstrate before and after changes with treatment (Figs. 10.2–10.4) (30). Having such a device in one's

Table 10.2 Body Contouring Baseline Documentation and Suggestions

Weight
Circumferential measurements, assisted by laser levels (Fig. 10.2)
Standardized two-dimensional photographs (Figs. 10.2 and 10.3)
  Use foot placement mats to guide distance from camera and posturing
  Use fixed lighting fixtures
  Capture front, and bilateral 45°, and 90° images
  Use same color background for all images
  Same undergarments (physician-provided disposable garments are helpful)
Standardized three-dimensional imaging (Fig. 10.4)
Laxity evaluation
  Skin punch
  Caliper
  Biomechanical tissue characterization

armamentarium helps to confirm the benefits of treatment for patients who may otherwise have only subjective feeling of improvement. It also acts as valuable protection in cases where patients claim inefficacy when progress has actually been achieved.

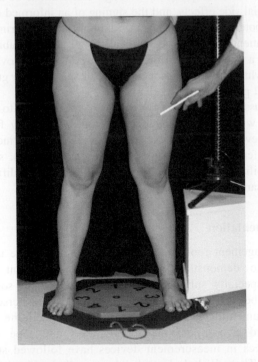

Figure 10.2 Standardized assessments, incorporating laser levels, foot placement mats, fixed lighting fixtures, simple black background, and consistent physician-provided undergarments.

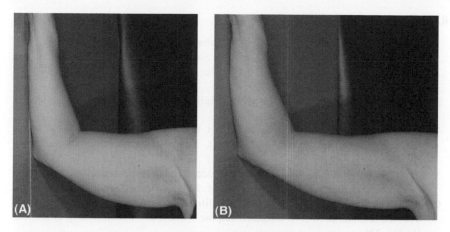

Figure 10.3 Standardized assessments, incorporating fixed lighting fixtures and apposition of an arm against a designated area of the wall for steadiness and consistency. The arm shown here is before (**A**) and 3 months after (**B**) treatment with a combined infrared, radio frequency, vacuum, and mechanical massage treatment regimen.

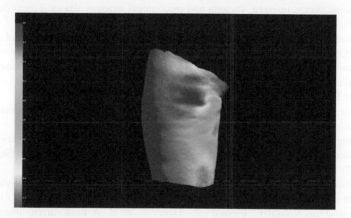

Figure 10.4 Three-dimensional objective imaging highlighting areas of consistency and change using color on a posterior thigh (image taken using the Vectra Imaging System, Canfield, Fairfield, New Jersey, U.S.).

CONCLUSIONS

With a plethora of new technologies now on the market and currently in development, proper patient selection and a firm understanding of the risks and benefits of each body contouring technique are crucial to the success of the procedure. An extensive pretreatment consultation and proper documentation allow the physician to select the most appropriate therapy, if any, for a given patient.

REFERENCES

1. West TB, Alster TS. Improvement of infraorbital hyperpigmentation following carbon dioxide laser resurfacing. Dermatol Surg 1998; 24(6):615–616.
2. Coleman WP. Cosmetic Surgery of the Skin: Principles and Techniques. Philadelphia, PA: B.C. Decker, 1991.
3. Avram MM, Harry RS. Cryolipolysis for subcutaneous fat layer reduction. Lasers Surg Med 2009; 41(10):703–708.
4. Anolik R, Chapas AM, Brightman LA, et al. Radiofrequency devices for body shaping: a review and study of 12 patients. Semin Cutan Med Surg 2009; 28(4): 236–243.
5. Taub AF, Battle EF Jr., Nikolaidis G. Multicenter clinical perspectives on a broadband infrared light device for skin tightening. J Drugs Dermatol 2006; 5(8):771–778.
6. Adamo C, Mazzocchi M, Rossi A, et al. Ultrasonic liposculpturing: extrapolations from the analysis of in vivo sonicated adipose tissue. Plast Reconstr Surg 1997; 100 (1):220–226.
7. Palm MD, Goldman MP. Laser lipolysis: current practices. Semin Cutan Med Surg 2009; 28(4):212–219.
8. Brightman L, Weiss E, Chapas AM, et al. Improvement in arm and post-partum abdominal and flank subcutaneous fat deposits and skin laxity using a bipolar radiofrequency, infrared, vacuum and mechanical massage device. Lasers Surg Med 2009; 41(10):791–798.
9. Hexsel DM, Mazzuco R. Subcision: a treatment for cellulite. Int J Dermatol 2000; 39 (7):539–544.
10. Brandi C, D'Aniello C, Grimaldi L, et al. Carbon dioxide therapy in the treatment of localized adiposities: clinical study and histopathological correlations. Aesthetic Plast Surg 2001; 25(3):170–174.
11. Hexsel D, Serra M, Mazzuco R, et al. Phosphatidylcholine in the treatment of localized fat. J Drugs Dermatol 2003; 2(5):511–518.
12. Chang P, Wiseman J, Jacoby T, et al. Noninvasive mechanical body contouring: (Endermologie) a one-year clinical outcome study update. Aesthetic Plast Surg 1998; 22(2):145–153.
13. Trelles MA, Mordon SR. Adipocyte membrane lysis observed after cellulite treatment is performed with radiofrequency. Aesthetic Plast Surg 2009; 33(1):125–128.
14. Pierard-Franchimont C, Pierard GE, Henry F, et al. A randomized, placebo-controlled trial of topical retinol in the treatment of cellulite. Am J Clin Dermatol 2000; 1(6):369–374.
15. Sasaki GH, Oberg K, Tucker B, et al. The effectiveness and safety of topical PhotoActif phosphatidylcholine-based anti-cellulite gel and LED (red and near-infrared) light on Grade II-III thigh cellulite: a randomized, double-blinded study. J Cosmet Laser Ther 2007; 9(2):87–96.
16. Bank DE, Perez MI. Skin retraction after liposuction in patients over the age of 40. Dermatol Surg 1999; 25(9):673–676.
17. Zelickson BD, Kist D, Bernstein E, et al. Histological and ultrastructural evaluation of the effects of a radiofrequency-based nonablative dermal remodeling device: a pilot study. Arch Dermatol 2004; 140(2):204–209.
18. Alvarez N, Ortiz L, Vicente V, et al. The effects of radiofrequency on skin: experimental study. Lasers Surg Med 2008; 40(2):76–82.

19. Arnoczky SP, Aksan A. Thermal modification of connective tissues: basic science considerations and clinical implications. J Am Acad Orthop Surg 2000; 8(5):305–313.

20. Gunin AG, Kornilova NK, Vasilieva OV, et al. Age-related changes in proliferation, the numbers of mast cells, eosinophils, and cd45-positive cells in human dermis. J Gerontol A Biol Sci Med Sci 2011; 66(4):385–392 [Epub 2010, Nov 24].

21. Dao H Jr., Kazin RA. Gender differences in skin: a review of the literature. Gend Med 2007; 4(4):308–328.

22. Mauriege P, Imbeault P, Langin D, et al. Regional and gender variations in adipose tissue lipolysis in response to weight loss. J Lipid Res 1999; 40(9):1559–1571.

23. Ley CJ, Lees B, Stevenson JC. Sex- and menopause-associated changes in body-fat distribution. Am J Clin Nutr 1992; 55(5):950–954.

24. Smith SR, Lovejoy JC, Greenway F, et al. Contributions of total body fat, abdominal subcutaneous adipose tissue compartments, and visceral adipose tissue to the metabolic complications of obesity. Metabolism 2001; 50(4):425–435.

25. Yu SS, Grekin RC. Aesthetic analysis of Asian skin. Facial Plast Surg Clin North Am 2007; 15(3):361–365, vii.

26. Manstein D, Laubach H, Watanabe K, et al. Selective cryolysis: a novel method of non-invasive fat removal. Lasers Surg Med 2008; 40(9):595–604.

27. Patel G, Hawley R, Johnson C, et al. Exploring and evaluating options for body shaping. Skin Aging 2009; 17(9).

28. Fitzpatrick R, Geronemus R, Goldberg D, et al. Multicenter study of noninvasive radiofrequency for periorbital tissue tightening. Lasers Surg Med 2003; 33(4):232–242.

29. Lack EB, Rachel JD, D'Andrea L, et al. Relationship of energy settings and impedance in different anatomic areas using a radiofrequency device. Dermatol Surg 2005; 31(12):1668–1670.

30. Weiss ET, Barzilai O, Brightman L, et al. Three-dimensional surface imaging for clinical trials: improved precision and reproducibility in circumference measurements of thighs and abdomens. Lasers Surg Med 2009; 41(10):767–773.

11

Nutrition, diet, and exercise

Ron Overberg

INTRODUCTION

It is often stated that diet and exercise are an important part of prevention and treatment of excessive weight and obesity. However, most insurance companies will not pay for people to receive nutrition counseling prior to getting obese and needing surgery. On the other hand, insurance companies will pay for and, in fact, insist that an obese patient should have three to six months of nutrition counseling prior to scheduled gastric bypass surgery. Thus, physicians end up being the primary source of information on nutrition and diet for their patients.

BACKGROUND

Often all that gets checked by a physician is patient's weight and body mass index (BMI); however, that may not be enough to uncover patients with poor nutrition and lifestyle habits. Patients may have an excellent BMI but still have no muscle tone, resulting in flabbiness. Water weight can compensate for muscle loss caused by lack of calories or protein in the diet. For example, a patient may have poor muscle tone in the upper body but a great tone in the legs. This is often seen in patients who accumulate water in their lower body, which keeps the skin tight and gives the appearance of well-toned legs. The burden of determining the need for nutrition and lifestyle counseling rests on the physician encountering the patient.

This chapter is based on my experiences with patients who experienced failure after having had a surgical procedure. It may be a very small percentage of the patients, but I only see the failures. Thus, the goal of this chapter is to increase the success rate of surgical procedures and to reduce adverse outcomes through nutritional support.

CLINICAL MANAGEMENT

Asking the Right Questions

From the 2010 Dietary Guidelines for Americans, "Poor diet and physical inactivity are the most important factors contributing to an epidemic of overweight and obesity affecting men, women, and children in all segments of our society. Even in the absence of overweight, poor diet and physical inactivity are associated with major causes of morbidity and mortality in the United States. Therefore, the Dietary Guidelines for Americans, 2010 is intended for Americans ages 2 years and older, including those at increased risk of chronic disease" (1).

Although this is true for the population of the Unites States as a whole, I have found the questions or points below to be instrumental in uncovering potential problems with each individual patient. Each question is designed to offer a clue as to the patient's likelihood of maintaining long-term good health and his or her ability to recover after a surgical procedure:

1. "Would you describe your eating patterns as poor? Are you skipping meals or have malabsorption issues?" This is one of the most common reasons that patients are seen for problems with postsurgical recovery; this is also an excellent tool to predict whether a patient is going to have such problems. Alternatively, the patient may fill out a dietary intake sheet and bring it to the appointment. In reality, however, few patients will comply.

2. It may be easier to walk the patient through the last 24 hours by asking the following questions: "What did you have for dinner last night? What time was that? Is that what you usually have? When did you go to bed? When did you get up? Did you sleep well? What did you have for breakfast? Is that what you usually have? What did you have for lunch? Did you have anything to drink? When did you eat next? Did you have a snack?" These questions have to be quite specific because many people associate eating with breakfast, lunch, and dinner and think that snacking in-between those meals does not fall under the category of eating. Thus, it may be helpful to ask "What did you have for dinner? Did you have something after dinner? What did you eat before you went to bed?"

3. These questions lead into an inquiry into food preferences. For example, if meat, milk, dairy, or fats are not mentioned, it may beg the following questions: "Are you vegetarian? Are you on a special diet (e.g., low-fat or no-fat)? Do you avoid particular foods (soy, eggs, and peanuts)? Do you have food allergies? What oils do you cook with and use in salad dressing?"

4. Next, the patient's support structure is explored. Questions that may be helpful to uncover those structures are "Who does the shopping? Who does the cooking? How many other people are in the household? If single and living alone, do family and friends bring food in or help with meal preparation?"

Answers to these questions may indicate many important issues with nutrition and, subsequently, chances of recovery. Skipping meals, especially breakfast, leads to a lower metabolism, since the body has no ready calories to burn. During lunch, this lower metabolism is not up to the task of digesting the meal, often resulting in postprandial drowsiness. Also, skipped meals often result in overeating at the next meal. In this way, a lower metabolism leads to a slow and steady weight gain if food intake is not adjusted accordingly.

Eating after dinner, eating before going to bed, or having dinner two to three hours before going to bed results in weight and fat gain due to insufficient time to metabolize the food. However, in certain cases, such as diabetic patients, a small late-night snack can stabilize blood sugar for a longer time.

Vegetarians are at risk for low levels of the following nutrients: vitamin B_{12}, carnitine, eicosapentaenoic acid (EPA) and docosahexaenoic acid (DHA), zinc, taurine, lipoic acid, conjugated linoleic acid (CLA), and iron. Carnitine, found in red meats, is needed for fatty acid transport into the mitochondria for energy production (2). CLA is found in milk products and is associated with weight loss.

People on no-fat diets will have issues with dry skin; a clue would be the use of lotions and lubricants all over the body. Often patients who use only olive oil in their diet will also report dry skin, because a balance of fats is needed for healthy skin. Thus, a proper diet should include some omega-3 oils (e.g., fish oil), omega-6 oils (e.g., safflower, sunflower, sesame, peanut, and soybean oils), omega-9 oils (e.g., olive, macadamia, and nut oils), and even some saturated fats.

A food intake history is especially important before follow-up visits. Often, those who do not progress as expected do not eat well. Patients may feel too tired as the day progresses and skip an evening meal. They may also be too tired to get up in the morning and have breakfast. They barely make it out the door for their appointment only to tell the practitioner that everything is going fine. Thus, direct questioning is often required and may reveal, for example, that they have not had anything since lunch the day before or only had a bowl of dry cereal for supper.

Formulating a Nutritional Plan

Caloric Intake

A rough yet very useful estimate of patient caloric requirements is comparison with the practitioner's own intake. For example, a patient who is one-half the size of the practitioner should consume about one-half the amount of food. If a patient exercises more than the practitioner, he or she will need to consume more calories. Although it's a rough guess, this allows the practitioner to uncover malnutrition, in terms of both quantity and quality of foods.

As an example from my own practice, a patient who wanted to eat ice cream every night was also extremely afraid of getting fat. To maintain her weight, she counted her calories, subtracted her ice cream calories from that amount, and reserved the rest for her nutritional needs. However, she did not eat enough food to nourish her body and was on one antidepressant after another. Her intake was too low, with most of the protein being used for calories. Thus, there was not enough L-tryptophan left in her diet to make serotonin. Therefore it would not matter what selective serotonin reuptake inhibitor (SSRI) she would be prescribed. Same could be said of dopamine, norepinephrine, and epinephrine, all of which are made from the amino acid L-tyrosine.

PROTEIN INTAKE

Apart from caloric intake, it is important to evaluate a patient's protein intake. A simple estimate is as follows: a portion of meat of the size of a deck of cards, such as a chicken breast, weighs approximately 3 to 4 oz (85–113 g). Most patients need about three "decks of cards" per day. Roughly, an ounce of meat contains about 5 g of protein, 1/2 cup of beans or grains contains 3 g, one slice of bread contains about 2 g, and a cup of milk or yogurt contains about 8 g. Animal meat, fowl, fish, shellfish, dairy, and eggs are common sources of complete proteins. Sources of incomplete proteins include legumes (beans and peas), which are low in methionine, and grains, nuts, and seeds, which are low in lysine. That is why well-trained vegetarians typically combine beans and grains in their dishes.

When educating a patient on adequate protein intake, the role of proteins and amino acids as building blocks throughout the body has to be emphasized (Table 11.1). Because of such varied functions in the organism, protein deficiency may have different manifestations, such as anemia, hair loss, chronic infections, poor muscle strength, and depression.

The recommended daily allowance (RDA) of protein is 50 to 60 g. However, it is important to remember that the RDA is an estimate for an average healthy person. Patients who have health issues such as chronic wounds, poor digestion, or are physically very active may require much higher amounts of

Table 11.1 Various Functions of Dietary Protein

Red blood cells and hemoglobin
White blood cells and antibodies
Enzymes, including digestive and metabolic (e.g., carbonic anhydrase)
Antioxidants, such as glutathione, metallothionein, and superoxide dismutase
Hormones
Neurotransmitters (e.g., serotonin from tryptophan; dopamine; norepinephrine and
    epinephrine from tyrosine)
Albumin (regulation of water balance)
Structural (e.g., hair, nails, skin, muscles)
Energy source, especially during starvation

protein. Since protein can also be used for energy, inadequate caloric intake will result in inability to properly heal and repair the body.

FRUIT AND VEGETABLE INTAKE

To roughly estimate the fruit and vegetable intake, each ½ cup of these foods counts for about one serving. If more precision is desired, a cup of leafy vegetables, such as salad leaves, counts as one serving, whereas ½ cup of mashed potatoes is considered a whole serving. A medium-sized fruit or vegetable (the size of a tennis ball) or 6 to 8 oz of real fruit or vegetable juice counts as a serving. No matter which technique is used, every nutritional survey appears to have the same result: very few people—between 5% and 10%—are getting the recommended amount of five servings of fruit and vegetables on a daily basis (and that is counting French fries and ketchup as two vegetables!).

Although all fruits and vegetables have a host of beneficial nutrients to offer and are a major dietary source of vitamin C, those with dark green, red, orange, and yellow insides offer even more benefits. Good examples of such fruits and vegetables include blueberries, red tomatoes, bell peppers, carrots, oranges, yellow squash, green spinach, and lettuce. These colors indicate high amounts of carotenoids and flavonoids, which have cardioprotective, free radical–scavenging, antiaging, and immunoprotective functions, thought to be mediated through increased natural killer cell activity and decreased lipid oxidation (3–5).

Carotenoids are a family of more than 600 fat-soluble antioxidants and include β-carotene. Fruits and vegetables rich in these chemicals include apricots, butternut squash, cantaloupe, carrots, grapefruit, greens, spinach, strawberries, and tomatoes. Cooking releases more of the carotenoids from the vegetable fibers. Also, consuming fat with these vegetables improves the absorption of carotenoids. On the other hand, juicing the vegetables and tossing the fiber reduce the amount of carotenoids.

The water-soluble antioxidants are the flavonoids, a family with more than 6000 members divided in flavones, flavanols, flavanones, anthocyanins, and catechins. Sources rich in flavonoids include apples, beets, berries, endive, French beans, grapefruit, green tea, kale, leeks, lemons, oranges, pears, and red wine. These chemicals reduce the risk of some cancers and heart disease, enhance immune function, and have anti-inflammatory action (6).

The third group of vegetables is the cruciferous family and includes broccoli, Brussels sprouts, cabbage, collard greens, horseradish, kale, mustard, radish, turnips, and turnip greens. These may help to protect against some malignancies, including gastric and lung, and, likely, breast, colon, and bladder cancer (7–11). According to the United States Department of Agriculture (USDA), on the average, Americans eat one serving of these vegetables per week instead of per day (12). Inhabitants of the United Kingdom fare slightly better with three cruciferous servings per week, but still miss the "one-a-day" mark (13). On the other hand, populations with some of the lowest breast and prostate cancer rates consume, on the average, eight servings of the cruciferous vegetables per week.

As demonstrated by the previous discussion, the greater the variety of fruits and vegetables being consumed, the better the overall health-protective benefits. However, people who frequently eat out never do well in the fruit and vegetables department, while excelling in the excess calorie, carbohydrate, and fat department. This is because fresh fruits and vegetables spoil rather quickly and then cannot be sold anymore. On the other hand, inexpensive, low-nutritional-value foods, such as green beans, coleslaw, and potato salad look good all day long and are favorite staples of restaurants. To drive this point home for patients, I recommend eating only white and yellow foods to age faster or, alternatively, eating a wide variety of colored fruits and vegetables to help them live longer.

ADDITIONAL CLINICAL CONSIDERATIONS

It is important to establish the patient's transit time, not just the regularity of bowel movements. For example, how long does it take for corn to appear in stool after being consumed at dinner? The longer it takes food to pass through, the more is absorbed, including hormones and cholesterol, despite a good intake of fiber. A transit time of 16 to 24 hours, facilitated by adequate fiber intake, is optimal for absorption of nutrients and is associated with lower risk of colon cancer, diverticulitis, and hemorrhoids (14–16). If bowel movements are not regular or are sluggish, a small dose of magnesium may help significantly.

Sleeping habits affect overall well-being nutrition, as well as recovery following trauma or procedures. The following questions may be asked: "How long do you sleep? How often do you wake up? Do you wake up because you have to go to the bathroom? How long does it take you go back to sleep? Do you feel refreshed when you wake up?" Apart from good sleep hygiene, such as sleeping in a totally dark room and abstaining from stimulating activities in the hours prior to bedtime, the following nutrients may help patients sleep better: calcium (500 mg at bedtime), magnesium (200–400 mg), melatonin (1–3 mg), L-tryptophan (500 mg), or phosphatidyl serine (100–300 mg). These supplements help patients fall asleep faster, sleep deeper, stay asleep, and wake up refreshed.

MEDICATION HISTORY

In my practice, I frequently encounter patients with rare side effects from various medications. Very often, the prescribing physician does not recognize the connection between a medication and a specific rare side effect, as numerous other patients in his or her practice have never experienced similar issues. Nonetheless, many clues may be picked up during patient interview if proper medication history is taken.

Adequate water intake is imperative for numerous medications that are eliminated by the kidneys. On the other hand, dietary fat and stomach acid are needed to trigger the release of bile, which is necessary for those medications that are metabolized by the liver. Overall, eating enough food is important as it stimulates the metabolism and, therefore, aids in the elimination of medications. Also, exercise stimulates circulation and elimination and also raises metabolism. All these factors are important to prevent medication overdose and to reduce the incidence of side effects. Consequently, various patient types may be at risk, including the elderly, the sedentary, the very thin and skinny, the very heavy, and the undereaters.

A good example of the complex interaction of medications, nutrition, and mineral homeostasis is long-term use of proton pump inhibitors and acid blockers. The body uses gastric acid to release vitamin B_{12} from food particles; decreased absorption may occur with long-term use of proton pump inhibitors and may lead to vitamin B_{12} deficiency (17). In addition, gastric acid is also needed to release minerals from food. Consequently, long-term use of these medications also results in hypomagnesemia (18). But magnesium is by no means the only mineral that can be deficient. The list also includes iron, calcium, boron, molybdenum, manganese, and chromium (19). In addition, gastric acid is also necessary to unfold proteins for their subsequent breakdown and for auto-catalytic cleavage of pepsinogen to pepsin, a major digestive proteolytic enzyme. Gastric acid also sterilizes food, while the combination of acid, protein, and fat in chyme triggers the release of secretin and cholecystokinin, which then regulate pancreatic and gallbladder function (20).

As can be seen from the previous discussion, the use of these medications compounds the nutritional deficiencies of patients already on a poor diet. The saving grace for many is that they overeat and, even though the percentage of minerals and other nutrients is reduced, they make up for it in volume consumed. Such patients will generally slowly gain weight, because they absorb proportionally more of the carbohydrates. The elderly, the chronically ill, the undereaters, and the weight-conscientious calorie counters are the ones in which such side effects are most common.

LABORATORY WORKUP

Several laboratory tests are important in determining the nutritional status of patients and to uncover nutritional deficiencies. Fasting glucose is used as a screen for prediabetic state or hypoglycemia. A patient may say: "My spouse tells me that if I don't eat on time, I become a bear to deal with." This is a person who has trouble switching from the carbohydrate-burning mode to fat-burning mode. Including enough protein and some fat in the diet along with carnitine and B-complex supplementation is very helpful in such cases.

Patient's cholesterol level should be determined, together with family history, to evaluate for the risk of heart disease. Lipoprotein particle testing is the best cholesterol and high- and low-density lipoprotein (HDL and LDL, respectively) evaluation. Additional testing for serum homocysteine, high-sensitivity C-reactive protein (CRP), fibrinogen, and lipoprotein(a) is recommended, as elevated levels are associated with a higher risk of heart disease even with normal cholesterol levels (21–24). Although rarely discussed, low cholesterol is also a concern. It should, however, come as no surprise that younger and younger men are featured in the advertisements for erectile dysfunction medications. Cholesterol is necessary for the synthesis of cortisol, a stress hormone needed to deal with the demands of life, but at the same time for the synthesis of testosterone and estrogens. Something has to give when cholesterol levels are too low.

Hypertriglyceridemia, with triglyceride levels more than 100 mg/dL, will make it harder for patients to lose weight. Also, it indicates one of several nutritional scenarios: overeating, an imbalanced diet with too many carbohydrates, or difficulty burning calories for fuel to maintain energy throughout the day. Apart from adjusting the diet, fish oil supplementation is helpful in such cases (25,26). Carnitine is another nutrient that aids in fat metabolism and may help to lower serum lipids (27–29).

Inflammatory markers, including sedimentation rate, CRP, and high-sensitivity CRP (hsCRP), tend to decrease with such simple nutrients as multivitamins, α-tocopherol (present in whole grains), omega-3 oils (cold-water fish), vitamin D (cod liver oil), carotenoids, curcumin (found in turmeric), and resveratrol (grapes) (30–36).

It is essential to test for serum 25-hydroxy vitamin D. Without adequate vitamin D, no amount of calcium will prevent osteoporosis; in addition, this vitamin has a positive impact on depression, heart disease, and weight control (37,38). Low serum phosphorus relative to calcium and low total iron-binding capacity (TIBC) are often associated with poor digestion and low protein absorption.

Complete blood count (CBC) can uncover numerous nutritional deficiencies or problems with absorption. A low mean corpuscular volume (MCV) can indicate a need for pyridoxine (vitamin B_6) and iron, whereas a high value can be seen with low folic acid and vitamin B_{12}. A high red blood cell distribution width (RDW) can also indicate a need for iron and vitamin B_{12}.

Additional useful tests to order are serum uric acid; γ-glutamyltransferase (GGT); alanine aminotransferase (ALT); aspartate aminotransferase (AST); and a complete iron panel including serum iron, TIBC, percent saturation, and serum ferritin. GGT is a more sensitive marker of liver damage than either AST or ALT, especially in alcohol-induced liver disease. As an indicator of iron storage, ferritin can often reveal previously undiagnosed hemocromatosis and is also an acute-phase reactant.

On the other hand, some deficiencies that have been going on for a long time will not show on blood tests until they become critical. For example, osteoporosis occurs despite normal serum calcium levels. The same is true for magnesium, as serum concentration is maintained at the expense of magnesium in muscle and other cells. Thus, the only test that will show a magnesium deficiency is the 24-hour urine magnesium load test.

VITAMIN AND MINERAL SUPPLEMENTATION

In addition to a standard multivitamin regimen, supplementation with several vitamins, minerals, and other nutrients is recommended (Table 11.2). Of importance, starting a magnesium supplementation program does not require low serum levels; instead, the following signs and symptoms should be sought out: cramps, spasms, tics, tremors, and twitches. Magnesium is an essential cofactor to make ATP and has more than 300 functions in the body, including bone health. It may also make a difference for patients who are irritable, sensitive to noise, anxious, short-tempered, or unable to concentrate and those who have excessive perspiration, rapid or irregular heartbeat, or who tend to wake up in the middle of the night. In general, patients who eat few leafy green vegetables, eat refined and

Table 11.2 Suggested Basic Vitamin/Mineral Supplementation

Vitamin/Supplement	Dose/Frequency	Notes
Multivitamin	Daily	With iron: younger than 20 years, anemia, females with monthly cycles Without iron: everyone else
Calcium	Male: 600–1000 mg/day Female: 600–1500 mg/day	Less if patient consumes dairy products
Magnesium	Male: bowel tolerance or 400–600 mg/day Female: bowel tolerance or 400–800 mg/day	Divided throughout the day, at least with breakfast and dinner or at bedtime
Fish oil	1—3 capsules/day	180 EPA, 120 DHA per capsule
Vitamin D	2000 IU (50 µg)/day	
Vitamin B complex	Suggested for those with low energy, usually at breakfast and lunch	Avoid supplementation at dinner because of stimulating potential
Vitamin C	500–4000 mg/day	Especially in patients recovering from surgery; best when spread throughout the day
Vitamin E	400 IU (136 tocopherol equivalents)/day	Especially in patients using many oils
Vitamin K$_2$, especially in the MK-7 form	40–80 µg/day	In patients with no green vegetables in their diet

processed foods, or consume large quantities of acid-forming foods such as coffee, carbonated drinks, meats, and grains may benefit from magnesium (39). It is recommended that the supplementation be divided into several doses per day to utilize magnesium more effectively and to delay the onset of diarrhea, one of its very few side effects. Caution should be exercised in patients with kidney failure, high-degree AV heart block, or a history of struvite kidney stones.

EXERCISE

Exercise is essential to maintain lean body mass in addition to the benefits for cardiovascular health. Muscle mass and strength decreases 30% to 50% between the ages of 30 and 80 years (40). Together with lost muscle mass, fat-burning capacity decreases with age. Cardiovascular exercise is important; however, all of the work is done by the legs. Thus, two to three hours of cardiovascular workouts per week are recommended, at a pace where the patient is still able to carry on a conversation. To be more precise, the proper pace should maintain the pulse rate at between 65% and 80% of 220 minus the patient's age. For example, a 50-year-old patient needs to keep his or her heart rate between 110 and 136 beats per minute.

Weight training and resistance exercises raise the overall muscle mass and tone the body with increasing weights. For adequate weight training, the weight should be heavy enough to make the 15th repetition difficult to perform with good strict form. Following two minutes of rest to allow the muscles to recover and rebuild ATP, the exercise is repeated with the same amount of weight. This time, only 12 to 14 repetitions are typically possible with good strict form throughout the exercise. Repetitions should be stopped when a good form cannot be maintained. Following another two minutes of rest, next exercise is undertaken using the same pattern.

A personal trainer is recommended at first to teach the correct form for each piece of exercise equipment and to reduce the risk of injury. Two weight-training sessions are recommended per week, ideally set 48 hours apart. On the first day, the workout concentrates on the chest, shoulders, triceps, and biceps, whereas the frontal thighs, hamstrings, and back are exercised on the second day. A light warm-up set is essential before exercising each body part, followed in the end by stretching (41).

Patients may start out by walking daily until they get in the habit of setting aside some time in their busy schedule for exercise. Following that, two days are typically devoted to weight training, as presented previously, while three or four days are dedicated to walking or other cardiovascular exercise.

CONCLUSION

Since nutrition counseling is generally not paid for by insurance companies and is rarely provided by physicians, more patients than necessary experience adverse outcomes after surgical procedures. This makes physicians the gate keepers to recommend nutrition evaluation and potential counseling to their patients. As can be seen from the previous discussion, nutrition evaluation is important and not difficult to incorporate into one's practice. Adding good nutrition to a surgical treatment produces the best outcome for the patient and saves time, money, and frustration for all involved.

REFERENCES

1. United States Department of Agriculture, Dietary Guidelines for Americans, 2010 (Released January 1, 2011) OMB 0584-0535. Available at: www.dietaryguidelines. gov. Accessed June 3, 2011.
2. Stephens FB, Constantin-Teodosiu D, Greenhaff PL. New insights concerning the role of carnitine in the regulation of fuel metabolism in skeletal muscle. J Physiol 2007; 581(pt 2):431–444.
3. Dixon ZR, Burri BJ, Clifford A, et al. Effects of a carotene-deficient diet on measures of oxidative susceptibility and superoxide dismutase activity in adult women. Free Radic Biol Med 1994; 17(6):537–544.
4. Dixon ZR, Shie FS, Warden BA, et al. The effect of a low carotenoid diet on malondialdehyde-thiobarbituric acid (MDA-TBA) concentrations in women: a placebo-controlled double-blind study. J Am Coll Nutr 1998; 17(1):54–58.
5. Kramer TR, Burri BJ. Modulated mitogenic proliferative responsiveness of lymphocytes in whole-blood cultures after a low-carotene diet and mixed-carotenoid supplementation in women. Am J Clin Nut 1997; 65(3):871–875.
6. Gullett NP, Ruhul Amin AR, Bayraktar S, et al. Cancer prevention with natural compounds. Semin Oncol 2010; 37(3):258–281.
7. Kim MK, Park JH. Conference on "multidisciplinary approaches to nutritional problems." Symposium on "nutrition and health." Cruciferous vegetable intake and the risk of human cancer: epidemiological evidence. Proc Nutr Soc 2009; 68(1): 103–110.
8. Meeran SM, Patel SN, Tollefsbol TO. Sulforaphane causes epigenetic repression of hTERT expression in human breast cancer cell lines. PLoS One 2010; 5(7): e11457.
9. Zhang CX, Ho SC, Chen YM, et al. Greater vegetable and fruit intake is associated with a lower risk of breast cancer among Chinese women. Int J Cancer 2009; 125(1): 181–188.
10. Kronbak R, Duus F, Vang O. Effect of 4-methoxyindole-3-carbinol on the proliferation of colon cancer cells in vitro, when treated alone or in combination with indole-3-carbinol. J Agric Food Chem 2010; 58(14):8453–8459.
11. Tang L, Zirpoli GR, Guru K, et al. Intake of cruciferous vegetables modifies bladder cancer survival. Cancer Epidemiol Biomarkers Prev 2010; 19(7):1806–1811.
12. Dixon ZR, Shie FS, Warden BA, et al. Effect of low carotene diet on malondialdehyde (MDA) concentration. FASEB J 1996; 10:A240.
13. Fenwick GR, Heaney RK, Mullin WJ. Glucosinolates and their breakdown products in food and food plants. Crit Rev Food Sci Nutr 1983; 18(2):123–201.
14. Burkitt DP. An epidemiological approach to gastrointestinal cancer. CA Cancer J Clin 1970; 20(3):146–149.

15. Burkitt DP, Walker AR, Painter NS. Effect of dietary fibre on stools and the transit-times, and its role in the causation of disease. Lancet 1972; 2(7792):1408–1412.

16. Burkitt DP, Walker AR, Painter NS. Dietary fiber and disease. JAMA 1974; 229 (8):1068–1074.

17. Ito T, Jensen RT. Association of long-term proton pump inhibitor therapy with bone fractures and effects on absorption of calcium, vitamin B12, iron, and magnesium. Curr Gastroenterol Rep 2010; 12(6):448–457.

18. Hoorn EJ, van der Hoek J, de Man RA, et al. A case series of proton pump inhibitor-induced hypomagnesemia. Am J Kidney Dis 2010; 56(1):112–116.

19. Insogna KL. The effect of proton pump-inhibiting drugs on mineral metabolism. Am J Gastroenterol 2009; 104(suppl 2):S2–S4.

20. Guyton AC, Hall JE. Textbook of Medical Physiology. 9th ed. Philadelphia: Saunders, 1996:825–829.

21. Sarwar AB, Sarwar A, Rosen BD, et al. Measuring subclinical atherosclerosis: is homocysteine relevant? Clin Chem Lab Med 2007; 45(12):1667–1677.

22. Pfutzner A, Forst T. High-sensitivity C-reactive protein as cardiovascular risk marker in patients with diabetes mellitus. Diabetes Technol Ther 2006; 8(1):28–36.

23. Okwuosa TM, Greenland P, Lakoski SG, et al. Factors associated with presence and extent of coronary calcium in those predicted to be at low risk according to Framingham risk score (from the multi-ethnic study of atherosclerosis). Am J Cardiol 2011; 107(6):879–885.

24. Katsouras CS, Tsironis LD, Elisaf M, et al. Lipoprotein(a) as a cardiovascular risk factor. Future Cardiol 2005; 1(4):509–517.

25. Guo W, Xie W, Lei T, et al. Eicosapentaenoic acid, but not oleic acid, stimulates beta-oxidation in adipocytes. Lipids 2005; 40(8):815–821.

26. Mori T, Kondo H, Hase T, et al. Dietary fish oil upregulates intestinal lipid metabolism and reduces body weight gain in C57BL/6J mice. J Nutr 2007; 137(12): 2629–2634.

27. Crayhon R. The Carnitine Miracle: The Supernutrient Program That Promotes High Energy, Fat Burning, Heart Health Brain Wellness and Longevity. New York: M. Evans, 1998.

28. Muller DM, Seim H, Kiess W, et al. Effects of oral ʟ-carnitine supplementation on in vivo long-chain fatty acid oxidation in healthy adults. Metabolism 2002; 51(11): 1389–1391.

29. Wutzke KD, Lorenz H. The effect of L-carnitine on fat oxidation, protein turnover, and body composition in slightly overweight subjects. Metabolism 2004; 53(8): 1002–1006.

30. Church TS, Earnest CP, Wood KA, et al. Reduction of C-reactive protein levels through use of a multivitamin. Am J Med 2003; 115(9):702–707.

31. Devaraj S, Leonard S, Traber MG, et al. Gamma-tocopherol supplementation alone and in combination with alpha-tocopherol alters biomarkers of oxidative stress and inflammation in subjects with metabolic syndrome. Free Radic Biol Med 2008; 44(6):1203–1208.

32. Eschen O, Christensen JH, LA Rovere MT, et al. Effects of marine n-3 fatty acids on circulating levels of soluble adhesion molecules in patients with chronic heart failure. Cell Mol Biol (Noisy-le-grand) 2010; 56(1):45–51.

33. Ginanjar E, Sumariyono, S, Setiati S, et al. Vitamin D and autoimmune disease. Acta Med Indones 2007; 39(3):133–141.

34. Morimoto T, Sunagawa Y, Fujita M, et al. Novel heart failure therapy targeting transcriptional pathway in cardiomyocytes by a natural compound, curcumin. Circ J 2010; 74(6):1059–1066.
35. Yang Y, Wang X, Zhang L, et al. Inhibitory effects of resveratrol on platelet activation induced by thromboxane a(2) receptor agonist in human platelets. Am J Chin Med 2011; 39(1):145–159.
36. Bereswill S, Munoz M, Fischer A, et al. Anti-inflammatory effects of resveratrol, curcumin and simvastatin in acute small intestinal inflammation. PLoS One 2010; 5(12):e15099.
37. Barnard K, Colon-Emeric C. Extraskeletal effects of vitamin D in older adults: cardiovascular disease, mortality, mood, and cognition. Am J Geriatr Pharmacother 2010; 8(1):4–33.
38. Cheng S, Massaro JM, Fox CS, et al. Adiposity, cardiometabolic risk, and vitamin D status: the Framingham Heart Study. Diabetes 2010; 59(1):242–248.
39. Houston M, Fox B, Taylor N. The Multifaceted Solution in What Your Doctor May Not Tell You About Hypertension. New York: Warner Books, 2003:45–88.
40. Frischknect R. Effect of training on muscle strength and motor function in the elderly. Reprod Nutr Dev 1998; 38(2):167–174.
41. Sheats C. Lean Bodies Total Fitness. Arlington, Summit Publishing, 1995:4–165.

12

Legal considerations

David J. Goldberg

INTRODUCTION

Legal considerations can arise in almost any aspect of an aesthetic practice. A full textbook on health care law would be required to adequately cover the varied legal issues as they relate to aesthetic treatments. This chapter focuses on the relationship between informed consent and the development of complications that may lead to a cause of action based on negligence. Since it is the lack of informed consent that may form the basis of a medical malpractice claim, the issues of what constitutes a medical malpractice claim will be fully described. Certainly there are different standards for a cause in medical malpractice throughout the world. This chapter focuses on the commonalities in medical malpractice.

BACKGROUND

The principle of informed consent establishes the patient's right to consent to a treatment or a procedure after being informed of the benefits or risks involved. The informed consent doctrine has three goals: (*i*) to include patients in the decision-making process; (*ii*) to involve the patient in values and choices that affect the social and physical aspects of life; and (*iii*) to ensure the patient is aware of the potential benefits and hazards of the treatment (1).

The informed consent doctrine would logically apply to patient approval of the procedure itself. In addition, such consent would also apply to any and all photographs and videotapes of the procedure. In complying with the principles of informed consent, a physician or other provider of treatment should notify the patient as to the benefits of the procedure as well as photography and videotaping. There is value to the use of such photography for teaching purposes, but the acquiescence to the videotaping and photos must come with appropriate patient consent.

THE STANDARD OF CARE

In general, in regard to medical care, a patient must be told all material issues that a reasonable medical practitioner would tell them. These principles can differ in concept in various jurisdictions, but in general the novice treatment provider would have to provide identical informed consent as would the more experienced physician. This is referred to as the "standard of care." Physicians are held to the "reasonable" standard of care. It would be reasonable for a physician to warn a patient about the risk of scarring from any energy or non-energy-based fat or cellulite treatment. It would not be the reasonable standard of care to warn a patient of a risk of death following antibiotic intake. Of course, what is reasonable is often determined by expert witness testimony. This standard of care will be similar for a dermatologist, plastic surgeon, or even aesthetician performing a procedure. If there is a breach in that standard of care leading to direct and proximate damages, the physician will usually be held liable in a malpractice case.

INFORMED CONSENT REQUIREMENTS

Although there are many potential causes of a physician malpractice case, the most common issue is the one of appropriate informed consent. It should be noted that consent could be either verbal or written. However, at the time of testimony in court, a signed patient document provides enormous credibility that the physician did give such consent. Appropriate signed consent is mandatory in today's litigious society.

Although initially the lack of informed consent in the United States was used to assert claims of assault and battery against physicians, today the lack of consent is at the very heart of medical malpractice claims based on negligence.

Complications do occur. They, in themselves, do not constitute medical malpractice. Whether a complication leads to a successful medical malpractice claim based on negligence lies in whether all the legal elements of cause of action, based on negligence, are fulfilled.

NEGLIGENCE

Any analysis of physician negligence must first begin with a legal description of the elements of negligence. There are four required elements for a cause of action in negligence. They are duty, breach of duty, causation, and damages. The suing plaintiff must show the presence of all four elements to be successful in his or her claim (1).

Defining the four elements of negligence, as relates to medical malpractice, is elusive but can be simply described as the following: (*i*) Duty is the conduct undertaken by another reasonable physician performing that very same treatment; (*ii*) a breach in that duty means the allegedly negligent physician did not undertake the treatment in the same manner as another reasonable physician undertaking the same treatment; (*iii*) causation refers to a connection between the breach in that duty and the fourth element of damages; (*iv*) damages are generally measured in terms of economic damages to the suing plaintiff, but may also refer to noneconomic damages such as emotional damages.

The duty of a physician performing fat, cellulite, and other noninvasive body-contouring procedures is to perform that surgery in accordance with the standard of care (2–4). Although the elements of a cause of action in negligence are derived from formal legal textbooks, the standard of care is not necessarily derived from some well-known textbook. It is also not articulated by any judge. The standard of care is defined by what an expert witness says it is and what a jury will believe. In a case against any dermatologist, the specialist must have the knowledge and have used the care and skill ordinarily possessed by a specialist in that field in the same or similar locality under similar circumstances. Any medical provider of a treatment will generally be held to an equal standard. A failure to fulfill such a duty may lead to loss of a lawsuit by the physician. If the jury accepts the suggestion that the physician mismanaged the case and that the negligence led to damage of the patient, then the physician will be liable. Conversely, if the jury believes an expert who testifies for the defendant doctor, then the standard of care in that particular case has been met. In this view, the standard of care is a pragmatic concept, decided case by case, and based on the testimony of an expert physician. The provider is expected to perform treatments in a manner of a reasonable physician. He or she need not be the best in his or her field; he or she need only perform the procedure in a manner that is considered by an objective standard as reasonable.

It is important to note that where there are two or more recognized methods of treatment, a physician does not fall below the standard of care by using any of the acceptable methods even if one method turns out to be less effective than another method. Finally, in many jurisdictions, an unfavorable result due to an "error in judgment" by a physician is not in and of itself a violation of the standard of care if the physician acted appropriately prior to exercising his or her professional judgment.

Evidence of the standard of care in a specific malpractice case includes laws, regulations, and guidelines for practice, which represent a consensus among professionals on a topic involving diagnosis or treatment, and the medical literature including peer-reviewed articles and authoritative texts. In addition, obviously, the view of an expert is crucial. Although the standard of care may vary country to country, it is typically defined as a "national" standard by the profession at large.

THE ROLE OF AN EXPERT WITNESS

Most commonly for litigation purposes, expert witnesses articulate the standard of care. The basis of the expert witness testimony—and, therefore, the origin of the standard of care—is grounded in the following: the witness' personal practice and/or the practice of others that he or she has observed in his or her experience, medical literature in recognized publications, statutes and/or legislative rules, and courses where the subject is discussed and taught in a well-defined manner.

The standard of care is the way in which the majority of the physicians in a similar medical community would practice. If, in fact, the experts do not practice like the majority of other physicians, then the experts will have a difficult time explaining why the majority of the medical community does not practice according to their ways.

It would seem then that in the perfect world, the standard of care in every case would be a clearly definable level of care agreed on by all physicians and patients. Unfortunately, in the typical situation, the standard of care is an ephemeral concept resulting from differences and inconsistencies among the medical profession, the legal system, and the public.

At one polar extreme, the medical profession is dominant in determining the standard of care in the practice of medicine. In such a situation, recommendations, guidelines, and policies regarding varying treatment modalities for different clinical situations published by nationally recognized boards, societies, and commissions establish the appropriate standard of care. In some of these cases, however, factual disputes may arise because more than one such organization will publish conflicting standards concerning the same medical condition. Adding to the confusion, local societies may publish their own rules applicable to a particular claim of malpractice. Certainly in the evolving area of fat, cellulite, and other body-contouring treatments, the standard of care itself is still evolving.

Thus, in most situations, the standard of care is neither clearly definable nor consistently defined. It is a legal fiction to suggest that a generally accepted standard of care exists for any area of practice. At best there are parameters within which experts will testify. A dermatologist's best defense is to act in accordance with the standard of care, to document appropriate risk assessment of the surgical patient, to provide appropriate medical record documentation and appropriate informed consent, and, finally, to use an appropriate treatment approach.

It is clear then that in order for the plaintiffs to win their negligence cause of action against any dermatologist, they must establish that their physician had a duty of reasonable care in treating them and had, in fact, breached that duty. However, that breach must also lead to some form of damages. A mere inconvenience to the plaintiffs, even in the setting of a physician's breach, will usually not lead to physician liability in a cause of action for negligence.

COMPLICATIONS VERSUS MEDICAL MALPRACTICE

It should be noted that the occurrence of a complication is not by definition medical malpractice. Laser- and radiofrequency-based thermal injuries can occur. However, when this happens, aggrieved patients often do seek legal advice. To lessen the likelihood of a lawsuit being filed, dermatologists must be very communicative with their patients. Plaintiffs file lawsuits for a variety of reasons. A patient who likes his or her doctor and can communicate with his or her physician is less likely to sue even when a complication has occurred. However, the best defense against a successful medical malpractice case, based on complications, is to be certain the dermatologist practices in accordance with the standard of care.

REFERENCES

1. Furrow BF, Greaney TL, Johnson SH, et al. Liability in Health Care Law. 5th ed. St. Paul, MN: West Publishing, 2004.
2. *Helling v. Carey.* 83 Wash2d., 514, Supreme Court of Washington, 1974.
3. *Gracey v. Eaker.* 837 So.2d., 348, Supreme Court of Florida, 2002.
4. *Velazquez v. Portadin.* 163 N.J., 677, 751, A.2d 102, Supreme Court of New Jersey, 2000.

Index

Page numbers followed by f and t indicate figures and tables, respectively.

Printed and bound by CPI Group (UK) Ltd, Croydon, CR0 4YY

18/10/2024

01776208-0001